# Cardiac Arrest

## What do you do?

*Also by the same author*
*The ECG – What does it tell?*

# Cardiac Arrest –
## What do you do?

**J. Gardiner, SRN, RCNT, RNT, Cert Ed (FE)**
Nurse Tutor, Gloucestershire College of Nursing and Midwifery

**Updated to include 1989 Resuscitation Council (UK) guidelines**

**Stanley Thornes (Publishers) Ltd**

# Cardiac Arrest – What do you do?

First published in 1986 by
Stanley Thornes (Publishers) Ltd
Old Station Drive
Leckhampton
CHELTENHAM GL53 0DN
England

Reprinted 1991 to include 1989 Resuscitation Council (UK) Guidelines

**British Library Cataloguing in Publication Data**

Gardiner, J.
    Cardiac arrest: what do you do?
    1. Heart failure   2. Medical emergencies
    3. Coronary care units
    I. Title
    616.1'29025     RC682

    ISBN 0–85950–243–0

Typeset in 10/12 Century Medium by Blackpool Typesetting Services Ltd
Printed and bound in Great Britain at The Bath Press, Avon

This book is dedicated to Sarah and all those who have tried.

# Contents

Preface                                                                    ix

Acknowledgements                                                            x

**Introduction**                                                           1
What is resuscitation?                                                     1
Why is resuscitation required?                                            1
Anatomy of the neck and chest                                             1
Respiratory arrest                                                        7
Cardiac arrest                                                            8
Causes of respiratory/cardiac arrest                                      8
Diagnosis – *effects of cardiac arrest – signs*                           10
Treatment                                                                 10

**Primary resuscitation**                                                 12
Airway – *clearing – maintenance*                                         12
Breathing – *expired air resuscitation (mouth-to-mouth, mouth-to-stoma,   15
        mouth-to-nose) – gastric distension*
Circulation – *history of cardiac massage/chest compression*             17
External chest compression (ECC) – *method – combined with expired air    20
                        resuscitation – common mistakes*
Precordial 'thump'                                                        25

**Secondary measures**                                                    26
Airway – *suction equipment – oropharyngeal airway – nasopharyngeal        26
        airway*
Breathing – *aids to expired air resuscitation – bag/value/mask units*    33

**Tertiary measures**                                                     36
Endotracheal intubation – *equipment – technique*                         36
Diagnosis of type of cardiac arrest – *The ECG*                           38

Defibrillation – *the need for defibrillation – technique of defibrillation – dangers of defibrillation – synchronised cardioversion*   40

Intravenous infusion   44

Resuscitation drugs   45

**Effects of cardiopulmonary resuscitation**   48

**Successful or?**   50

**Aftercare**   52

**Future developments in cardiopulmonary resuscitation** – *cough CPR*   53

**Appendixes**   54

Treatment of choking – *the Heimlich technique (abdominal thrust, chest thrust) – back blows*   54

Recovery position   63

Endotracheal intubation – *equipment – technique – oesophageal obturator airway*   66

Hypothermia   77

Paediatric resuscitation – *airway – breathing – circulation – ECG – defibrillation – drugs*   79

ECG recognition – *sinus rhythm – sinus bradycardia – sinus tachycardia – premature atrial contractions (atrial ectopics) – supraventricular tachycardia – premature ventricular contractions (ventricular ectopics) – R-on-T ectopics – ventricular tachycardia – ventricular fibrillation – ventricular standstill – ventricular flutter – asystole – third-degree heart block*   89

**Index**   113

# Preface

This book is intended to be of use to any individuals who may be involved in the resuscitation of those who have suffered respiratory and/or cardiac arrest.

It should be of particular use to ambulance personnel involved in the pre-hospital phase of patient care and to nurses, junior medical and paramedical staff involved in the in-hospital phase of patient care.

It has been updated in 1991 to include the 1989 Resuscitation Council (UK) guidelines.

Gloucester 1991                                                    J. GARDINER

# Acknowledgements

My thanks go to those who helped me in the production of this book. To Elaine, Mandie and Mike who helped with the diagrams and photographs; to the following organisations who lent me equipment for the diagrams and photographs:

Ambu International (UK) Limited

International Medication Systems (UK) Limited

Laerdal Medical Limited

Physio-Control Limited

and, most of all, to Sue for her encouragement.

# Introduction

## What is resuscitation?

Resuscitation is a means of sustaining life, of preventing deterioration and, ideally, of improving the patient's condition.

This usually consists of maintaining an adequate oxygenated supply of blood to the brain and other vital organs.

The methods of resuscitation used may vary from 'basic techniques' to more 'advanced techniques', they will vary from patient to patient and may include only airway-care in the unconscious patient, support of the circulation by fluid replacement or full cardiopulmonary resuscitation (CPR).

## Why is resuscitation required?

Damage occurs to a body that is deprived of oxygen, for even a short time. While some tissues may have some degree of recovery, the brain will die rapidly if deprived of oxygen (see Effects of cardiac arrest, page 10).

It is therefore vital that we find some means of imitating the circulation and function of the lungs if normal function has ceased. This must be continued until normal function is restored, to prevent brain damage or death.

## Anatomy of the neck and chest

In resuscitation the head and neck are important as they contain the brain and the upper airway. The brain is vital since the whole purpose of resuscitation is to maintain brain function, while the airway must be kept patent to ensure adequate flow of the oxygen-containing air to the lungs.

The chest contains the heart and lungs – important organs which enable oxygen to enter the circulation and to be transported around the body, particularly to the brain.

We will look in turn at the airway, breathing and circulation.

## Airway

The airway is the passageway through which air passes from the mouth/nose down to, but not including, the alveoli. Let us look at some problems that may affect the airway.

First we have a *dual system*. Air may enter either through the nose and nasal cavity to the *nasopharynx* or through the mouth, past the tongue to the *oropharynx* (Figure 1).

The two channels become one at the oropharynx and here we meet the first problem. The tongue is a large muscular organ attached to the lower jaw (mandible) and in the conscious individual is held well forward in the mouth. But if the individual should become unconscious the tongue becomes flaccid. If the patient is lying on his back, the tongue can easily fall backwards and totally block the airway (Figure 6, page 12). This will need to be remedied or the patient will die.

Continuing down the oropharynx we find that the passageway then divides

Figure 1. A cross-section of the head and neck to show the airway

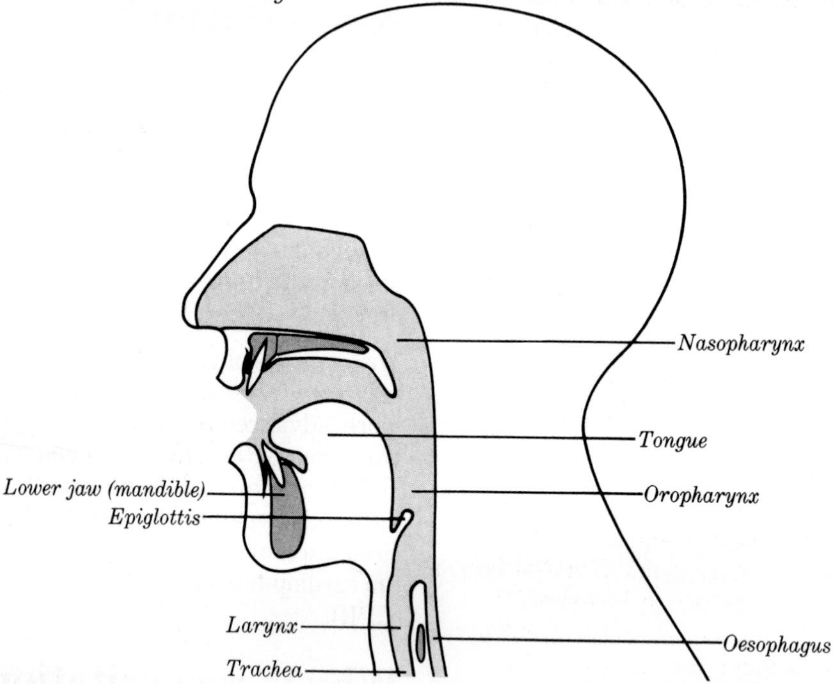

with the airway moving anterior in the neck, the air entering the *larynx*. The structure behind is the *oesophagus*, via which food may reach the stomach.
Obviously we need something to stop food entering the larynx – this is the *epiglottis*, a small flap which covers the entrance to the larynx when food/drink is swallowed. The epiglottis is found at the base of the tongue; the angle between the epiglottis and the tongue is known as the *vallecula*.

Occasionally the epiglottis fails in its function and allows food or drink to enter the larynx (often because we try to override the system by attempting to talk and swallow at the same time, but its function is also depressed and may be altogether absent in unconscious people or in patients in a state of cardiac arrest). At the entrance to the larynx are the *vocal cords*; if any foreign material touches these they may well go into spasm. Usually when foreign material enters the larynx in the conscious individual he coughs and ejects the object. Occasionally the object may pass the vocal cords and obstruct the airway. Once again urgent management is required to clear the obstruction. If the patient is unconscious he may be unable to cough in response to the stimulus and, instead, the airway will be obstructed (Figure 7, page 13).

Below the larynx, the air will pass down the *trachea*, which then divides at the *carina* into the right and left *bronchi* (Figure 2(a)). The left bronchus leaves the carina at a more acute angle than the right, and

*Figure 2(a). The lungs and pleura*

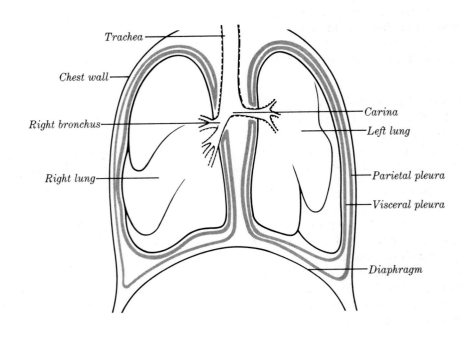

therefore any foreign material that gets this far usually enters the right bronchus and therefore enters the right lung.

When an endotracheal tube is passed (see Appendix 3, page 66), if it is too long it may well enter the right bronchus instead of stopping above the carina (Figure 2(b)).

Both bronchi subdivide into smaller and smaller *bronchioles* which eventually terminate as *alveoli*. Alveoli are sacs which have the appearance of bunches of grapes, and it is here that gas exchange takes place (Figure 3).

**Breathing**
To enable this gas exchange to take place (i.e. the movement of oxygen into the circulation and carbon dioxide back into the alveoli) there must be some method of moving the air in and out of the lungs.

*Figure 2(b). The endotracheal tube in position*

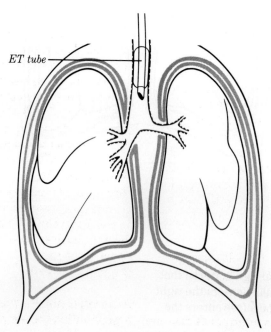

*Figure 3. An alveolus*

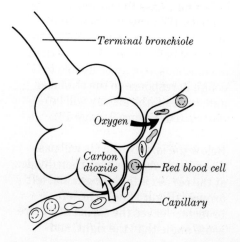

In the chest we have the trachea, bronchi and lungs. We also have the mechanics of respiration (Figure 2(a), page 3). These are:

(1) The *diaphragm* – a dome shaped muscle that forms the base of the chest cavity.
(2) The *pleura* – a double layered membrane; the outer (*parietal*) layer is attached to the chest wall and the inner (*visceral*) layer is attached to the lungs.
(3) The *chest wall* – the ribs, intercostal muscles, skin etc.

Normally the diaphragm contracts, flattening downwards, thus increasing the size of the chest cavity. Because the parietal pleura is attached to the diaphragm it moves down with it, and as there is a slight negative pressure between the two layers of the pleura (there is only a potential space between the two) the visceral pleura must follow the parietal. The lungs move, expand, with the visceral pleura and air is drawn in via the airway. There is also some contraction of the *intercostal muscles* with normal respiration, increasing the size of the *thoracic cavity*. The diaphragm and intercostal muscles then relax allowing the lungs to return to their resting position and air is passively exhaled.

If more air is required (e.g. during exercise) the individual can voluntarily expand the chest wall by contracting the intercostal muscles between the ribs and increase the size of the chest cavity even further and therefore expand the lungs even more.

The levels of oxygen and carbon dioxide in the blood are monitored by chemical receptors (*chemoreceptors*) sited in various parts of the body. Low oxygen or high carbon dioxide levels are therefore automatically assessed and the rate and/or depth of respiration adjusted accordingly (e.g. if you voluntarily hold your breath, at some point the body takes over – forcing you to breathe).

It should not be difficult to accept that it does not take any great problem to affect this system and make breathing difficult or impossible. If breathing does stop one merely has to blow air into the patient's lungs for them instead.

## Circulation

Oxygen is moved around the body via a system of arteries, capillaries and veins (Figure 4, page 6). The power for this movement is supplied by a muscular pump – the *heart* (Figure 5, page 7).

Oxygen enters the blood at the alveoli and this blood returns to the heart via the pulmonary veins. It enters the left *atrium* of the heart passing through a one-way valve (the *bicuspid or mitral valve*) into the left *ventricle*. This is the real workhorse of the heart as this chamber must pump the blood around the body. Blood leaves the left ventricle through another valve (the *aortic valve*) into the aorta and from this vessel it travels both up to the head (brain), shoulders and arms, and down to the rest of the body and legs (Figure 4, page 6).

After supplying the brain and other organs within the body with oxygen

5

Figure 4. Circulation

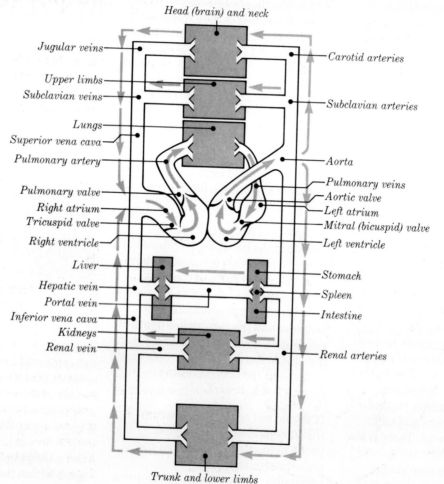

Head (brain) and neck

Jugular veins
Carotid arteries
Upper limbs
Subclavian veins
Subclavian arteries
Lungs
Superior vena cava
Pulmonary artery
Aorta
Pulmonary veins
Pulmonary valve
Aortic valve
Right atrium
Left atrium
Tricuspid valve
Mitral (bicuspid) valve
Right ventricle
Left ventricle
Liver
Stomach
Hepatic vein
Spleen
Portal vein
Inferior vena cava
Intestine
Kidneys
Renal vein
Renal arteries

Trunk and lower limbs

and picking up the waste carbon dioxide, the blood returns to the right side of the heart via the superior and inferior *venae cavae*. It then enters the right atrium and passes through the *tricuspid valve* into the right ventricle. From here it passes through the *pulmonary valve* to the pulmonary arteries and back to the lungs (Figure 5).

The heart continues pumping from before birth until death; in the adult the rate is 70–80 beats per minute (b.p.m.). If the heart should fail to pump blood, for any reason, death will follow quickly and it becomes essential that the function of the heart and circulation are taken over by artificial means for the individual to have any chance of survival.

# Respiratory arrest

This occurs when insufficient air is moved to and from the lungs (usually with no or negligible movement) to supply oxygen to the body and remove carbon dioxide from it.

Normally a reduction in the partial pressure of oxygen ($pO_2$) or an increase in the partial pressure of carbon dioxide ($pCO_2$) in the blood will result in an increase in the rate and/or depth of respiration. But if the disease process or trauma present prevents this or there is physical damage to the mechanics of respiration (see Causes of respiratory/cardiac arrest, page 8), the level of oxygen in the lungs (alveoli) and blood will diminish.

The low $pO_2$ will affect the body generally and the brain in particular, stopping the normal aerobic metabolism. Anaerobic metabolism may commence but this is inefficient and results in the production of acid metabolites (e.g. pyruvic and lactic acids). These further depress body function.

*Figure 5. The heart*

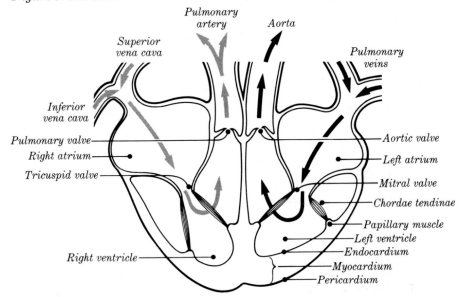

7

This *acidosis*, together with the continuing lack of oxygen, can readily produce cardiac arrest, and also make resuscitation difficult.

# Cardiac arrest

By definition this is:
<u>an inability of the heart to maintain an adequate cerebral circulation in the absence of a causative or irreversible disease.</u>

This may sound long-winded but simply indicates that the heart has stopped functioning or is not functioning as it should, thus resulting in a loss of cardiac output. Because of this loss, the supply of blood, and therefore oxygen to the brain stops. The brain has no reserves of oxygen, and within minutes of this loss occuring, damage will be incurred.

The phrase 'in the absence of a causative or irreversible disease' suggests that cardiac arrest is a potentially reversible situation if treated correctly and promptly. Also that if the patient has died of 'natural causes' or following irreparable trauma it may not be appropriate to attempt resuscitation. Normally this decision would be made by a doctor. If a decision has not been made prior to the cardiac arrest or if there is any doubt, it may be better to commence resuscitation, continuing the attempt until a decision can be made or until the rescuer is physically unable to continue the resuscitation attempt.

Both cardiac arrest and respiratory arrest can occur separately depending upon the initial cause. But, if one occurs and treatment is not implemented quickly, the other will follow, e.g. if a patient has a respiratory arrest and is left, his heart will also stop functioning.

# Causes of respiratory/cardiac arrest

The causes are many and varied, some will cause both respiratory and cardiac arrest at the same time, others will only cause one or the other to occur.

Ideally, by removing or treating the cause and initiating resuscitation the respiratory/cardiac arrest will be reversed.

It may be difficult or impossible to treat or remove the cause, or it may be dangerous to approach the patient (e.g. one who has been electrocuted) or, of course, the patient may have succumbed to an irreversible or terminal disease. In this case, it may be impossible/difficult/dangerous to attempt resuscitation and it may become a question of whether one should attempt resuscitation or not. (See Successful or?, page 50.)

The causes may be divided into the areas of the body which they affect:

### Airway

The commonest cause of airway obstruction is the tongue falling back in the unconscious person and this may be easily remedied (see Figure 6, page 12 and Appendix 2, page 63).

Alternatively inhalation of a foreign body (e.g. food or a toy) may obstruct the airway (see Figure 7, page 13 and Appendix 1, page 54). Also local swelling may occur following an insect sting, burns, scalds, effects of corrosives on the airway etc. Plastic bags, pillows or similar soft material may occlude the mouth and nose and so prevent entry of air (*suffocation*). The airway may also be compressed from outside the neck, due to hanging or strangulation.

## Larynx

Spasm may cause constriction within the larynx resulting in a gross reduction of the amount of gases entering or leaving the lungs. Causes of this may include the inhalation of food, water, smoke or other irritant gases.

## Trachea/bronchi

These may be occluded by food or other foreign material.

## Bronchioles

The passage of air may be affected by the presence of spasm, or mucus as a result of asthma or bronchitis.

## Thoracic cavity

This may be affected by:
(1) Compression from outside as a result of a fall of sand, earth, grain etc., or any other heavy weight.
(2) Damage to the chest wall following trauma, which may include crush injury, flail segment, open wounds, rib fractures, ruptured diaphragm, etc.
(3) Trauma to the heart and/or lungs, e.g. pneumo- or haemothorax, tension pneumothorax, cardiac tamponade.
(4) Disease affecting the heart and/or lungs, e.g. spontaneous pneumothorax, myocardial infarction, pulmonary embolism.

## Central nervous system

Damage may be caused by:
(1) Electrocution.
(2) Trauma – head injury, spinal cord injury.
(3) Disease – polio, tetanus, cerebrovascular disease.
(4) Poisoning – accidental or non-accidental, toxic gases, chemical agents, drug overdosage, animal poisons (anaphylactic reaction).
(5) *Hypoxia* (low oxygen level) – due to displacement of oxygen by carbon monoxide or non-toxic gases; due to airway obstruction; due to continuous grand mal fits (status epilepticus); due to major blood loss (loss of oxygen carrying capacity).

## Conduction system

Damage to the conducting tissue and a resulting dysrhythmia may be caused by:
(1) Electrocution.
(2) Overdose of drugs (e.g. digoxin).
(3) Ischaemic heart disease (e.g. myocardial infarction).

It is possible to add more causes to the above list, but it should give some indication of the many causes of cardiorespiratory arrest.

As will be evident from some of the above causes, it may be of great importance to ensure the safety of the rescuer before approaching the patient (to prevent more than one requiring resuscitation).

9

The definition of cardiac arrest (page 8) suggests that it is potentially reversible but if the trauma received or the disease process present is irreversible, irreparable or terminal in nature, it may not be appropriate to attempt resuscitation.

# Diagnosis

To consider how to diagnose we must first consider the effect of oxygen deprivation on the brain and look at the signs produced by this.

### Effects of cardiac arrest

The partial pressure of oxygen ($pO_2$) in the cerebral blood vessels will drop to approximately one-fifth of what it normally is within 10 sec of the cessation of supply. This will result in a loss of conciousness.

The cerebral $pO_2$ will drop to zero within approximately 1 min resulting in respiratory arrest occurring (if this was not the precursor of the cardiac arrest). Irreversible brain damage occurs within minutes of this happening.

Also, as the blood flow to the tissues has ceased, there is general tissue hypoxia and a build-up of waste products, as they are not removed. This leads to several effects of which the most important is the lactic acidosis produced by the anaerobic metabolism.

### Signs

All these effects can lead to a number of signs that can be used to diagnose cardiac arrest. But of these there are two main signs that will always be present and these two alone are all that are required to diagnose cardiac arrest:

(1) Unconsciousness – ensure by verbal stimulus and/or physically shaking the patient, that he is actually unconscious and not asleep!
(2) No major arterial pulses (carotid or femoral pulse).

If these two signs are present then the patient is in a state of cardiac arrest. The other signs develop as the general tissue and cerebral hypoxia increase and irreversible brain damage occurs.

The other signs that may be seen are:

*Cerebral* – respiration ceases (just as respiratory arrest will lead to cardiac arrest if untreated), although the patient may initially gasp for a short period of time; pupils dilate and will become unresponsive to light.

*General* – pallor or greyness (other colours may be seen depending upon the cause of arrest, e.g. carbon monoxide poisoning – cherry red);
   – cyanosis may or may not be present, may be central and/or peripheral;
   – cold, clammy skin.

# Treatment

This can be roughly divided into three stages (primary, secondary and tertiary), depending on the expertise of the operator and the amount/standard of equipment/personnel available.

But all should:
(1) Care for the patient's airway.
(2) Support the patient's respiratory state.
(3) Imitate the heart's action.

They should therefore maintain a supply of oxygenated blood to the vital organs, and may also, with a degree of luck, restore the normal action of the heart.

For the following we will assume that the patient is in a state of both respiratory and cardiac arrest.

# Primary resuscitation

Primary resuscitation consists of the basic A, B, C of resuscitation, i.e.,

A Airway – clear it and maintain it.
B Breathing – take over with artificial ventilation.
C Circulation – imitate the heart's action with external chest compression.

First ensure that your patient is unconscious and not merely asleep. Speak as you approach the patient. If there is no response, shake your patient gently whilst continuing to speak. If there is still no response from the patient, assume that there is some degree of impairment of the level of consciousness.

## Airway

In an unconscious patient lying on his back the flaccid tongue will fall back and obstruct the airway (Figure 6).

*Figure 6. The tongue occluding the airway*

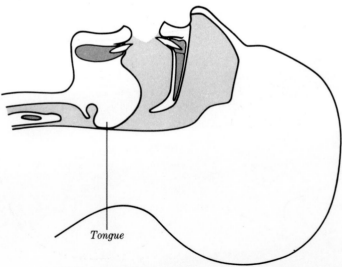

Tongue

Also the patient's airway may be contaminated with vomit or other foreign material (Figure 7) which may be the cause or result of the arrest. So this must be cleared and the patent airway maintained.

First sweep your fingers through the mouth, clearing any vomit, loose teeth, loose dentures or other foreign material (a handkerchief/tissue/ material may be wrapped around the fingers if necessary). To open the mouth a

'cross-finger' technique may be used, if the jaw is not tightly clenched. To use this technique, just push against the lower jaw/teeth with the thumb and the upper jaw/teeth with the forefinger of the same hand (Figure 8).

*Figure 7. A foreign body occluding the airway*

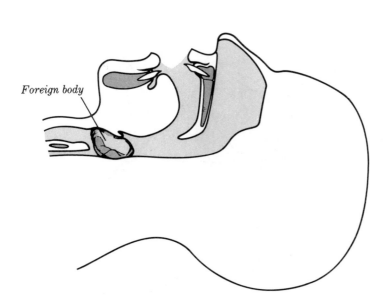

Foreign body

*Figure 8. Opening the mouth – cross-finger technique*

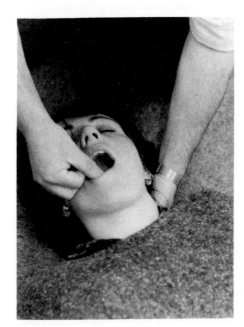

If dentures are firmly in position they may be left in place to aid the seal of lips when mouth-to-mouth ventilation is attempted. If the dentures are loose or it is only a partial plate, the dentures may be removed to prevent the risk of them becoming dislodged and entering the airway.

Next we must stop the tongue from obstructing the airway. This is best attempted by extending the patient's neck, thus pulling the jaw and with it the tongue forward to clear the airway.

To accomplish this stand/kneel level with the patient's neck/shoulders. The hand nearest to the patient's chest should be placed under the patient's neck, near to the back of the head, and the other hand on the patient's forehead. The hand under the neck is lifted and the hand on the forehead pushes the head back (Figure 9). This lifts the lower jaw up and forward, pulling the tongue with it to clear the airway, while the mouth also tends to open a little.

If the patient was suffering from a respiratory arrest because of obstruction of the airway and this has

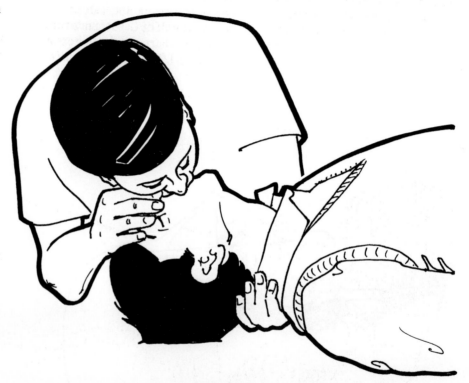

*Figure 9. Mouth-to-mouth ventilation*

now been cleared, he may then gasp and attempt to breathe. If breathing becomes adequate, place the patient in the recovery position (see page 63, Appendix 2). If breathing is not adequate or the patient is not breathing at all, then initiate expired air resuscitation.

14

If the patient vomits again, turn the head to one side to allow drainage of the vomit. If necessary place the patient on his side in a head-down position to permit drainage of the vomit.

# Breathing

There are various methods of *artificial ventilation* (without any equipment) of which the one usually taught, and the most efficient, is *expired air resuscitation* – EAR (mouth-to-mouth or mouth-to-nose ventilation). (See Figures 9 and 10.)

First ensure that the patient is not breathing or that breathing is so inadequate that assistance is required. Having cleared/checked the airway, place your cheek near the patient's mouth. You should be able to feel breath on your cheek, hear the air movement and see movement of the chest (Figure 11). If you do not feel, hear or see this, breathing is not adequate or is totally absent.

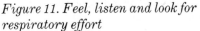
*Figure 10. Mouth-to-nose ventilation*

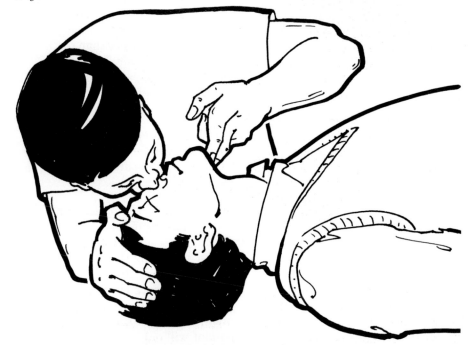

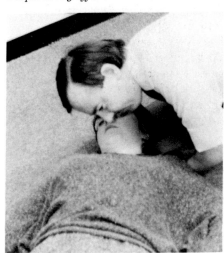
*Figure 11. Feel, listen and look for respiratory effort*

## Mouth-to-mouth ventilation

Once you have extended the neck you will have one hand under the patient's neck and one on his forehead. Leave the one under his neck and, keeping the heel of the other hand on the forehead (or top of the nose), pinch the patient's nose with the fingers of that hand (Figure 12).

*Figure 12. Airway extended, nose occluded – prior to mouth-to-mouth ventilation*

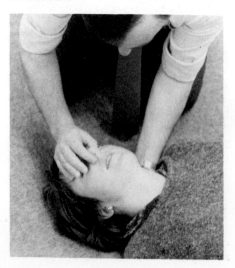

Place your lips over the patient's (completely sealing the patient's mouth) and exhale into the patient. Watch for chest movement when you exhale. If you feel a lot of resistance to your breath and/or the chest does not move, extend the neck a little more as the tongue may still be obstructing the airway. If you are still unable to inflate the lungs, ensure that you have a complete seal over the patient's mouth and that there is no leak from the nose. If still unsuccessful, sweep around the mouth again with your fingers and try to inflate the lungs again.

It may be worthwhile checking the front of the patient's neck for a tracheostomy. If a tube or just an opening (stoma) is found, commence ventilation by placing your mouth over the tracheostomy.

In the patient who has had a laryngectomy this may be sufficient to inflate the chest. If the patient only has a temporary tracheostomy there may be a leak of air back out of the mouth and nose. If so, cover and seal the mouth and nose with one hand, leaving the other under the neck.

If there is no tracheostomy and ventilation attempts are still unsuccessful, it may be because there is a complete obstruction of the airway. Attempt to clear it using the Heimlich technique (see Appendix 1, page 54).

On seeing the patient's chest rise, move your face away from the patient's so allowing the patient to exhale passively and allowing you to obtain fresh air rather than the patient's exhaled air. There is also the risk that the patient may vomit. It may then be preferable to have your face away from the patient's.

You should observe the patient's chest falling as he exhales, therefore ensuring that you are ventilating the patient.

Initially inflate the patient's lungs with two slow breaths. At that point you may assess the patient's cardiac output by feeling the carotid pulse (Figure 15, page 20). If there is no pulse, commence external chest compression (page 20). If the pulse is present and is of good volume, the patient will only require ventilation.

Continue ventilating the patient at, approximately, the rate of once every 5 sec (12 times/min). Continue at this rate until the patient is breathing adequately for himself or until more efficient techniques/equipment are available.

Do not take deep breaths yourself and/or blow hard into the patient. If you hyperventilate, you will soon feel faint/dizzy and will be unable to continue ventilating the patient efficiently (or at all). Breathe only at a slightly deeper depth than normal if you are not moving the patient's chest very much. As long as there is obvious movement of the patient's chest you are ventilating the patient adequately.

## Mouth-to-nose ventilation

If you are unable to maintain a seal around the patient's mouth with your lips, e.g. when the patient's mouth is bigger than yours or the patient's mouth/lips have been damaged by trauma/corrosive chemicals, it may be more efficient/safer to use the mouth-to-nose method of expired air resuscitation.

Keep your hand on the forehead and bring the other from under the neck to the chin. Use this hand to lift the lower jaw toward the nose (keeping the lips together and helping to keep the tongue out of the airway) (Figure 10, page 15). Place your mouth over the patient's nose and exhale as with mouth-to-mouth ventilation.

When ventilating a small child it may be easier to cover the child's mouth and nose with your mouth and use less force when ventilating, just enough for the chest to rise (see Appendix 5, page 79).

## Gastric distension

Artificial ventilation may frequently cause gastric distension. It occurs most commonly in children, but is not uncommon in adults. It usually occurs when excessive pressures are used to ventilate the patient and/or the airway is partially obstructed and some air takes the 'easy' route into the oesophagus and stomach.

The risk of gastric distension is greatly reduced if only enough pressure is used to inflate the lungs to the point where the chest can be seen to rise.

Marked distension of the stomach may promote regurgitation and also reduce the lung volume by elevating the diaphragm.

If the stomach becomes distended during resuscitation, recheck and reposition the airway and continue artificial ventilation using reduced force.

Do not attempt to relieve the gastric distension by pressing the stomach. This may cause regurgitation of the gastric contents with a high risk of aspiration of these contents into the lungs. It may be difficult to prevent this occuring even if suction equipment is immediately to hand.

If regurgitation does occur whilst resuscitating the patient, quickly turn the patient onto his side and wipe out the mouth before continuing resuscitation.

# Circulation

So far we are keeping the patient's airway clear and we are getting oxygen into the patient's lungs, but we want to get that oxygen to the brain. So we must also take over the circulation if it is not functioning naturally.

The heart is situated relatively centrally in the chest with the sternum in front and spinal column behind (Figures 13 and 14), the lungs lie either side of the heart.

*Figure 14. A cross-section of the chest*

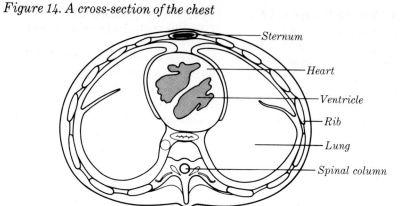

*Figure 13. The position of the heart and lungs in the chest*

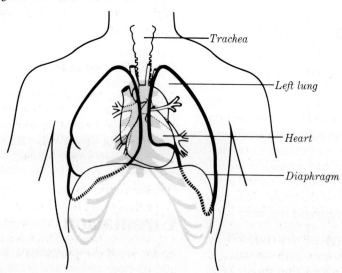

### History
Back as far as 1786 it was suggested that by compressing the sternum the circulation could be imitated. In 1874 experiments were performed in open chest cardiac massage and in 1885 Dr F. Koenig, in Germany, reported six successful resuscitation attempts in humans using external chest compression. But up until the 1960s it was usual for the chest to be opened to allow internal cardiac massage to be attempted. This was usually only performed successfully in the operating theatre.

In 1960 C.G. Knickerbocker and his colleagues at the Johns Hopkins Hospital found that sternal compression in dogs resulted in a carotid blood flow. At the same time W.B. Kouwenhoven and his colleagues combined the techniques of artificial ventilation, sternal compression and electrical defibrillation in the resuscitation of dogs and eventually humans.

So, at this time, the concept of external sternal compression became accepted. It was suggested, and readily accepted, that blood was pumped by squeezing the heart between the sternum and the spine (Figure 20, page 22), the valves in the heart ensure a one-way flow of blood. This theory has been taught by many organisations since and is accepted world-wide.

In 1976 Dr J.M. Criley in Los Angeles described a patient who remained conscious during an attack of ventricular fibrillation (page 53) simply by coughing repeatedly. Dr Criley suggested that the rise in pressure within the chest as a result of the coughing must have compressed the heart in some way.

A year later a study showed that it is important to 'squeeze' the chest during sternal compression and therefore the duration of compression became more important than the actual rate. A number of individuals were investigating the mechanism of chest compression and proposed that the heart did not function as a pump but that the whole chest did!

Dr L.A. Cobb in Seattle demonstrated that the valves of the heart did not actually move during compression and Dr Criley demonstrated that a valve-effect in the superior vena cava prevented a return of blood during compression and therefore helped in ensuring a one-way flow of blood.

Another group went on to show that an increase in intrathoracic pressure increased the circulatory output from the chest during compression (by ventilating at the same time as compressing). All this seemed to be fairly conclusive. Unfortunately, at the same time another group was able to disprove the chest compression theory and the idea of the heart as a pump continued to be accepted.

In 1982 a group under Dr S.J. Rankin in America went on to prove that the heart was 'squashed' during compression and that the valves did function. They also proved that the faster one compressed the chest (up to a rate of 150 compressions/min), the greater the output from the heart. Dr Rankin's group called this *high impulse cardiopulmonary resuscitation*.

## Where do we stand?

From all the work that has been published over the past few years it seems likely that both mechanisms are effective when cardiopulmonary resuscitation is undertaken.

At slow compression rates it would seem likely that the whole chest acts as a pump, whereas the smaller capacity heart works more efficiently as a pump if compressed much more rapidly.

19

*How does this affect the individuals involved in cardiopulmonary resuscitation in the practical setting?* It would seem unlikely that an individual could keep up a high rate of compression for any length of time, and it makes ventilation of the patient by expired air resuscitation very difficult. If expired air resuscitation is performed at the same time as external chest compression, air is more likely to enter the stomach and regurgitation may occur. Therefore it is suggested that the method described in the following section is practical. But once an endotracheal tube has been passed and a number of operators are available it may well be worth considering high impulse cardiopulmonary resuscitation if the senior doctor present decides it is worthwhile.

It is suggested that once an endotracheal tube has been passed and the cuff is inflated (see Appendix 3, page 66), it is no longer necessary to coordinate ventilation and sternal compression. If both happen to occur together, it may well result in an increase in cardiac output/carotid flow.

# External chest compression (ECC)

External chest (or cardiac) compression – ECC, is a means of maintaining the circulation by artificial means. A rhythmic compression of the sternum forces blood out of the chest, and it refills when the compression is relaxed.

Obviously, first there is a need to assess the pulse to ensure there is a need to support the circulation. Always check a major pulse, e.g. carotid or femoral: the carotid is often the most accessible (Figure 15), remember to palpate for a full five seconds. If a major pulse is not palpable, then assume there has been a circulatory collapse and commence external chest compression.

Your hands must be placed on the patient's chest over the sternum (Figure 16).

*Figure 15. Assess for the presence of a carotid pulse*

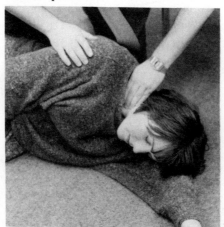

*Figure 16. The hand position for external chest compression*

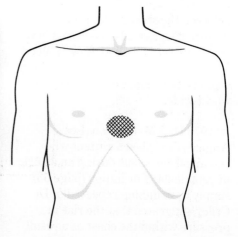

20

This is done by first identifying the lower end of the sternum by running your fingers up across the abdomen into the 'V' of the lower edge of the ribs. Three fingers of one hand (usually the hand that was nearest to the patient's feet) are placed on the sternum immediately above this point (Figure 17). The heel of the other hand is placed on the sternum immediately above the fingers (Figure 18). The heel of the first hand

*Figure 17. 'Three fingers up from the end of the sternum'*

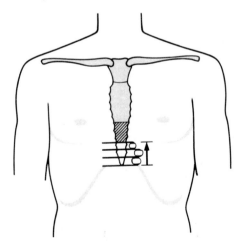

*Figure 18. The heel of the second hand is placed above the fingers of the first hand*

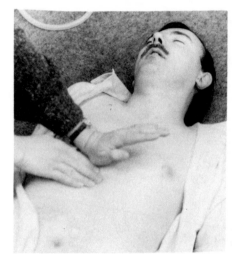

is now placed over the heel of the hand already in position.

At this point the heels of your hands are at the junction of the middle and lower thirds of the sternum (Figure 19) (in the male it will be noted that the hands lie on a line between the two nipples, in the young female the lower hand will apparently be cupping one breast).

The fingers, if possible, should be kept clear of the chest wall, if necessary the fingers may be intertwined. This ensures that any downward force is applied directly over the sternum and that the pressure is not spread over the chest

*Figure 19. Hands in position, arms straight; the weight of the upper body of the rescuer is transferred to the chest of the patient*

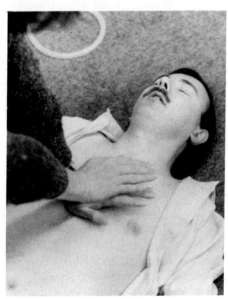

21

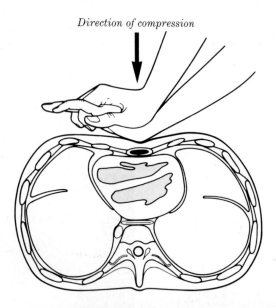

*Figure 20. A downward force is applied over the sternum*

Direction of compression

wall (wasting your energy and reducing the efficiency of ECC) (Figure 20).

Keeping your arms straight (Figure 19, page 21) (this is easiest if you are standing/kneeling very close to the patient's side) exert force directly down on to the sternum, using the weight of the upper part of your body.

A slight rocking motion is allowed as you take your weight off the patient (to allow the heart/chest to refill), but there should *not* be an obvious rocking movement as this may cause your weight to be pushed laterally across the chest wall, not straight down as is required.

The downward thrust should be delivered smoothly, not as a jerk, and should depress the adult sternum approximately $1\frac{1}{2}$ to 2 in (4 to 5 cm).

In the adult, external chest compression should be continued at a rate of approximately once per second, with the downward thrust occupying $\frac{1}{2}$ sec and the release $\frac{1}{2}$ sec. This rate may be maintained if the operator counts (to himself or out loud) 'one one thousand', 'two one thousand', 'three one thousand', etc. – compressing on the first single figure.

**Artificial ventilation with ECC**
If the patient needs artificial ventilation and ECC together, they are continued as follows:
If one person is resuscitating alone – initially give two ventilations, then 15 compressions and continue at a rate of 2 ventilations to 15 compressions (the ECC at a rate of 80/min). (When resuscitating alone the rate of ECC is greater than once per second.) Therefore count 'one *and two and three and four*', etc. compressing on

the number. Taking ventilation into account over the minute gives an average of 60 compressions per minute.

If two persons are resuscitating – after the initial two ventilations, one person continues ECC at a rate of 1 compression per second without pause. The other person must ventilate the patient, timing the ventilation to coincide with a pause between compressions (Figure 21).

*Figure 21. Two persons resuscitating*

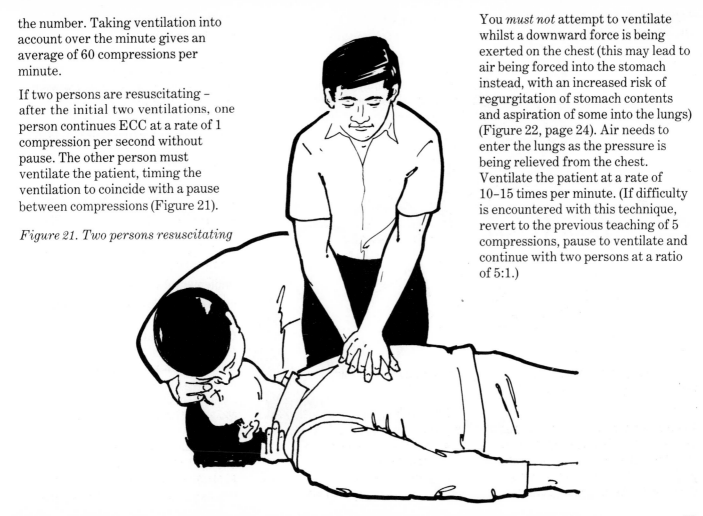

You *must not* attempt to ventilate whilst a downward force is being exerted on the chest (this may lead to air being forced into the stomach instead, with an increased risk of regurgitation of stomach contents and aspiration of some into the lungs) (Figure 22, page 24). Air needs to enter the lungs as the pressure is being relieved from the chest. Ventilate the patient at a rate of 10–15 times per minute. (If difficulty is encountered with this technique, revert to the previous teaching of 5 compressions, pause to ventilate and continue with two persons at a ratio of 5:1.)

23

*Figure 22. Do not ventilate whilst the chest is being compressed*

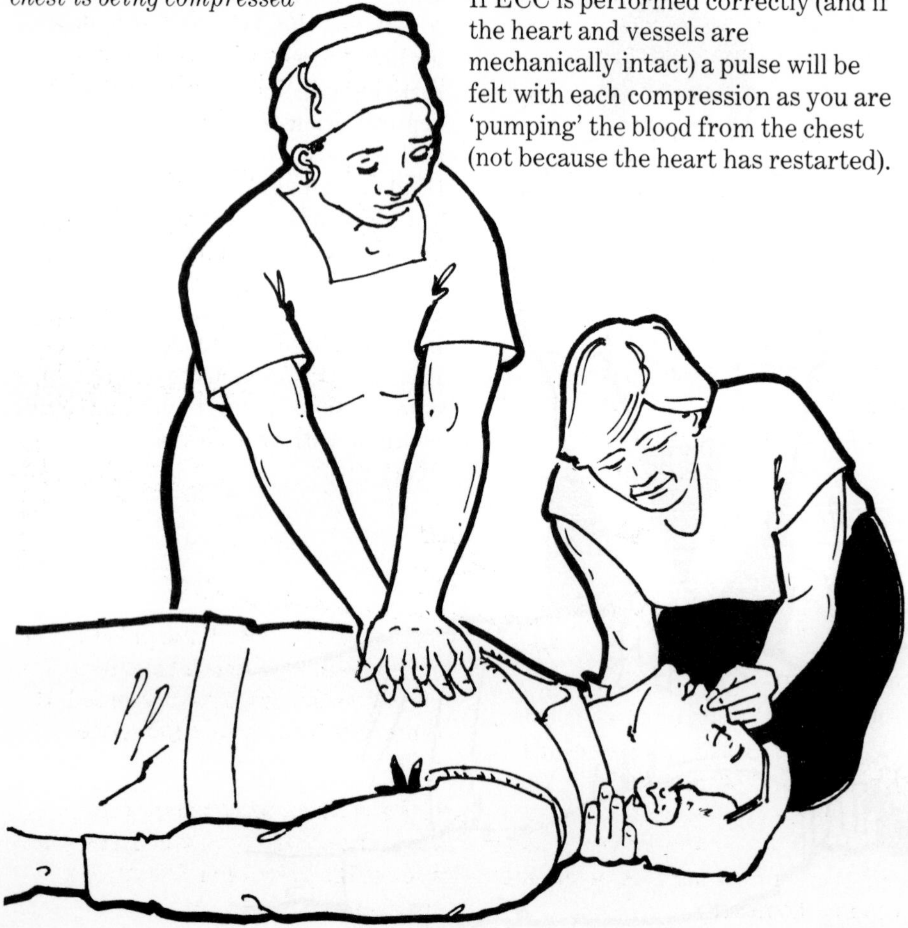

## Pauses in ECC

If ECC is performed correctly (and if the heart and vessels are mechanically intact) a pulse will be felt with each compression as you are 'pumping' the blood from the chest (not because the heart has restarted).

To find out if the heart has restarted stop ECC for 10–15 sec and check for a major pulse, if none is found within that time recommence ECC. This must be checked for after the first minute of resuscitation and at approximately 3–4 min intervals, or more often at the request of a doctor.

ECC should be continued until there is a return of cardiac output (i.e. a return of the pulse), with no pause in ECC of greater than 10–15 sec. A pause is only allowed to assess for the presence of a pulse, for the two personnel to swap around if the one performing ECC is tiring or for the implementation of one of the more advanced resuscitation techniques.

## Common mistakes

ECC if performed correctly is fairly efficient, but several common mistakes may occur:

*Rocking* – as already mentioned, the force exerted needs to be *straight down* on the chest not laterally across the chest wall.

*Bending the elbows* – thus less force gets to the patient and/or you have to work harder, so getting tired more quickly. Keep your arms *straight*.

*Thumping* – if your hands leave the chest wall each time you ease off the downward pressure, you waste time and energy obtaining contact with the chest wall again. Thus you tire more quickly and ECC is less efficient. Also your hand position may vary, with the risk that you will compress in the wrong position, adding the possible complication of rib fractures.

*Jerking* – sharp, short 'jerks' against the chest wall may look good but are not as efficient as steady smooth compressions and will result in a less efficient circulatory output.

*Hand position* – if the hand position is incorrect, ribs or the lower end of the sternum may be fractured resulting in damage to the lungs, heart, liver etc.

Occasionally when resuscitating the elderly patient (or any other patient with a 'stiff' chest) ribs may fracture even though the hand position is correct. If this occurs,

do not worry as the fractures are usually on the outer aspect of the rib cage and do not usually result in damage to internal structures.

Ensure that the position of your hands is correct and that the heels of your hands remain in contact with the patient's chest (over the junction of the middle and lower third of the sternum).

## WARNING
Do NOT practise expired air resuscitation or external chest compression on live patients, only on a training manikin with an instructor.

(For ECC in infants/children see Appendix 5, page 79.)

# Precordial 'thump'

If the patient is actually seen to collapse and is found to be pulseless, or you are assessing the pulse of a patient and it stops whilst you are counting it, i.e. you witness the cardiac arrest, it may be worth using one precordial 'thump' to attempt to restart the heart.

Using a clenched fist give the patient a good 'thump' at the point where you would place the heel of your hand for ECC (start off with your fist at a height of 12–18 in (30–45 cm) above the chest) (Figure 23).

*Figure 23. Precordial 'thump'*

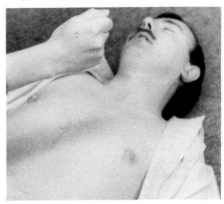

Following this, check the pulse again – if you feel a pulse you have been lucky and the heart has restarted. If there is still no pulse, commence ECC.

If there is any doubt about exactly when the cardiac arrest occurred, do not use the precordial 'thump' but commence ECC immediately.

# Secondary measures

These secondary measures are improvements on the initial measures and apply to airway care and ventilation. External chest compression remains the same.

## Airway

If the airway has been contaminated by blood or gastric contents it may not be totally cleared by sweeping a finger across the mouth, so suction equipment should be used as soon as it is available.

There are many types of equipment available – both portable and fixed appliances – working off compressed gas, batteries, mains electricity, a piped vacuum, or manually (usually using one's foot). It is up to the individual to obtain tuition on the equipment in his particular area (not only on how to use the equipment but also on how to clean it and prepare it for re-use). (Figures 24–27.)

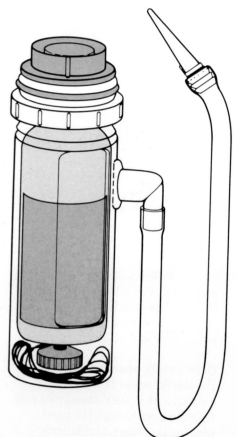

*Figure 24. Gas operated suction (Laerdal 'jet sucker')*

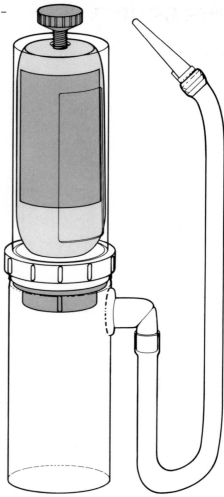

*Figure 26. The Laerdal 'jet sucker' – ready for use*

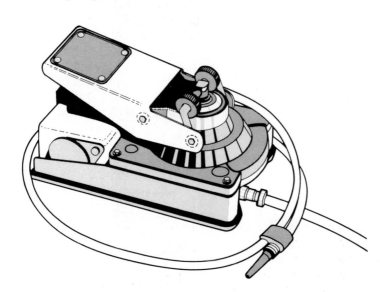

*Figure 25. Foot operated suction (Ambu suction 'pump')*

Figure 27. Battery operated suction
(Laerdal suction unit)

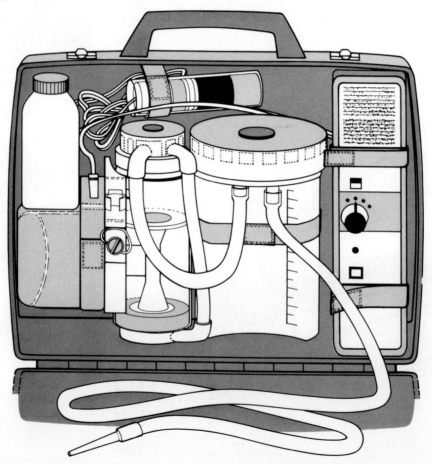

When aspirating the oropharynx it is usual to use a rigid suction catheter, e.g. a Yankaur catheter (Figure 28), except in small children and infants or when performing nasopharyngeal suction. In these a flexible suction catheter is easier to use and less traumatic.

It is wise to pass a rigid suction catheter only as far as you can see to minimise the risk of damage to the patient. Your view can be improved by opening the patient's mouth wide, either by using the cross-finger technique (page 13) or by using a laryngoscope. Obtain the best view

you can to enable you to clear the pharynx as much as possible.

One can also use a suction booster (Figure 29). This ensures a very high flow rate via a large bore catheter or via an endotracheal tube and sometimes may be all that will clear

*Figure 28. Use a rigid suction catheter when aspirating the oropharynx*

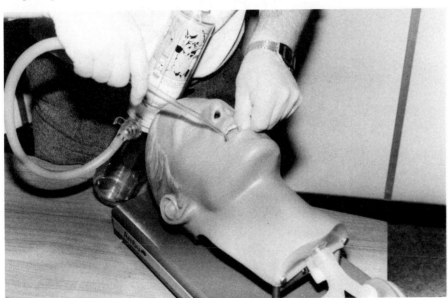

*Figure 29. Ambu suction booster*

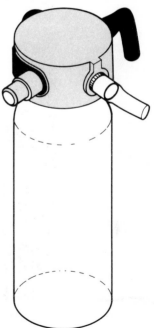

the airway adequately of a large volume of gastric contents or other fluid matter. To use it you connect your suction equipment to one outlet on the suction booster and the large bore catheter or an endotracheal tube to the large port. When the other small port is occluded with a finger, a vacuum is applied at the end of the suction catheter (Figure 30). The small reservoir may fill quickly but is very easy to empty.

To aid with the maintenance of the airway an oropharyngeal 'airway' (e.g. a Guedel airway) may be used. This is a curved rubber or plastic tube which has a metal reinforced piece and flange at one end. Its function is to separate the lips and teeth and to keep the tongue clear of the posterior pharyngeal wall (Figure 31).

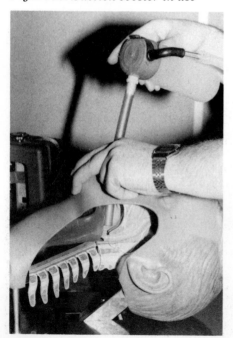

*Figure 30. Suction booster in use*

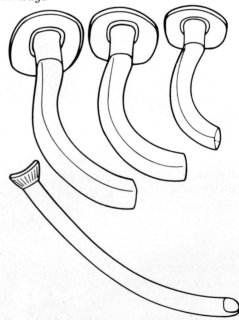

*Figure 31. Oropharyngeal and nasopharyngeal airways*

This helps to ensure a clear air entry and aids oropharyngeal suction, using a soft suction catheter alongside or through the oropharyngeal airway. The reinforced piece is kept between the teeth to stop the recovering patient from biting/damaging the airway. The flange outside the lips helps to maintain the oropharyngeal airway in the correct position.

Oropharyngeal airways are graded from the smallest at 000, getting progressively larger through 00 and 0, 1, 2, 3, to the largest, 4. Infants up to 1 year require 000 to 0. Children from 1 to 5 years require 0 to 1. From 5 years to puberty 1 to 2 (occasionally 3) is needed. Adults require from 2 to 4 depending upon overall size.

Correct choice of size is important, as too small an airway may not pass the flaccid tongue and too large an airway may have its opening occluded by the posterior pharyngeal wall or, more commonly, may cause retching/vomiting in the patient who is recovering consciousness. One can assess the approximate size required by comparing the airway chosen with the distance from the corner of the lips to the angle of the jaw of the patient.

To ensure that the oropharyngeal airway does not actually cause airway obstruction by pushing the tongue back, it should be inserted with the tip of the oropharyngeal airway pointing at the roof of the mouth (Figures 32 and 33). Once it is approximately $\frac{3}{4}$ of the way in it is

*Figure 32. Insertion of oropharyngeal airway*

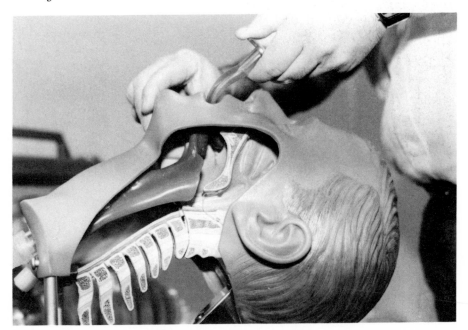

*Figure 33. Oropharyngeal airway being inserted*

rotated through 180° so that the tip of the oropharyngeal airway moves into position behind the tongue (Figure 34).

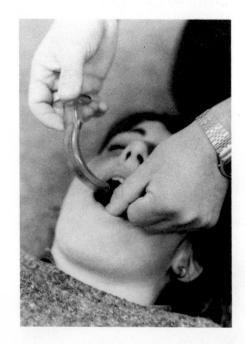

*Figure 34. Oropharyngeal airway* in situ

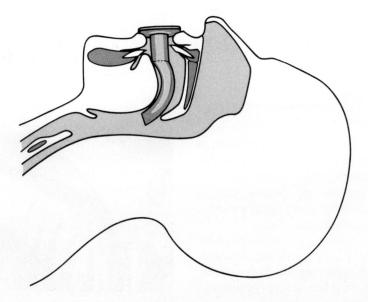

Also ensure that the lips are not trapped between the oropharyngeal airway and the patient's teeth. There should be an easy passage of air via the oropharyngeal airway.

Once consciousness is returning, if the patient starts to 'gag'/retch it is wise to withdraw the oropharyngeal airway slightly (approximately 1–2 cm). Upon recovery of consciousness allow/encourage the patient to remove the airway himself (by hand or, often, by pushing it out with his tongue). If the patient does it himself it ensures that he will then be able to maintain his own airway to a satisfactory degree.

As long as the patient accepts the airway one can assume that he needs it left *in situ*.

If it is difficult to use an oropharyngeal airway, e.g. because of local trauma, it may be possible to insert a nasopharyngeal airway instead. A nasopharyngeal airway looks like a short endotracheal tube (approximately 5 in (13 cm) long) with a flange, or it may be made by cutting short a non-cuffed endotracheal tube and putting a safety pin through the end of it (Figure 31, page 30).

The nasopharyngeal airway is introduced into a nostril (lubricate it first), and is passed back through the nasopharynx into the oropharynx, and therefore will help maintain the airway.

It is important to remember that the nasopharynx lies parallel to the roof of the mouth, therefore do NOT push the nasopharyngeal airway straight 'up the nose'. If there is any resistance do NOT push hard, turn the airway slightly and try again. If unsuccessful do not keep trying. In spite of being gentle there may be some bleeding and aspiration of this may be required using suction equipment.

Even with an oro- or nasopharyngeal airway *in situ* it will be necessary to keep the patient's head extended so as to ensure a patent airway. If you are unsuccessful in placing the oro- or nasopharyngeal airway in position do not waste time/effort by continuing to attempt insertion, but maintain the patient's airway by the methods already described.

# Breathing

Performing expired air resuscitation can be made more pleasant by using aids such as the 'Resusci-Aide', 'Pocket Mask', or the 'Brook airway'. These minimise contact between rescuer and patient which may be particularly useful if there is the risk of infection from the patient.

The Brook airway is an instrument that has an oropharyngeal airway at one end which is placed in the patient's mouth; a flange then covers the mouth. Above the flange is a one-way valve and the operator can blow into the airway, and therefore the patient, knowing that the patient's exhaled air will exit from the side of the one-way valve. The airway can be easily disassembled for cleaning.

The efficiency of ventilation can be improved by using a bag/valve/mask unit such as the 'Ambu bag' or the 'Laerdal Resuscitator' (Figures 35 and 36). This is because you are then using normal room air to ventilate the patient and not your exhaled air. Exhaled air contains only 15–16% oxygen, compared to 21% in room air.

When using a bag/valve/mask unit it is easier if you stand or kneel behind the patient's head, facing down the body. After the patient's airway has been cleared, the head/neck can be extended by the following: place one hand on the patient's forehead and the fingers of the other hand under the tip of the patient's jaw, pull back on the jaw and push down on the forehead.

Keep the head/neck extended with your fingers under the jaw and place the mask over the patient's nose and mouth (it will be found that the mask is narrower at one end, this end is placed over the nose). The mask is held in position by placing your thumb over the nose part of the mask and first finger over the mouth part.

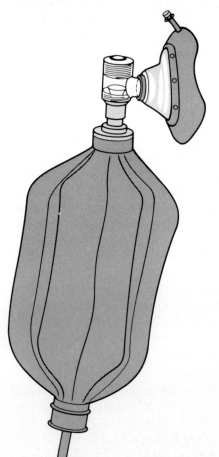

*Figure 35. An Ambu compact resuscitator*

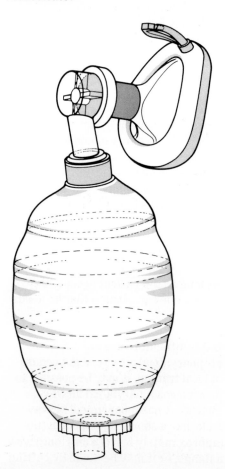

*Figure 36. A Laerdal adult resuscitator*

These should push down, maintaining a seal on the patient's face. The rest of the fingers on that hand are kept under the jaw and by pulling back on these the neck/head is kept extended (Figure 37).

*Figure 37. The neck/head is kept extended*

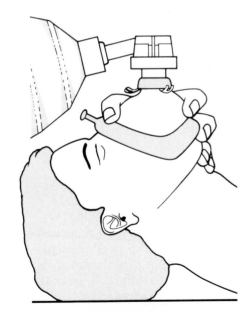

The other hand that was on the forehead is now available to squeeze the bag (Figure 38). If your hand is too small to squeeze the bag easily, it can be compressed between your hand and the patient's head or against your side if you are close enough to the patient.

If available, oxygen may be added via the inlet on the back of the bag/valve/mask unit. Some units give the option to enable the operator to administer 100% oxygen during the resuscitation procedure, e.g. the oxygen reservoir bag on the 'Laerdal resuscitator'.

If one person is still attempting resuscitation alone it may be performed more efficiently if that person continues with the measures mentioned under Primary resuscitation (page 12).

Suction will have helped to improve the care of the airway but too much time is wasted trying to use a bag/valve/mask unit after every 15 compressions. (The position of the operator alongside the patient needs to be different when performing

EAR and ECC to that when using a bag/valve/mask unit).

The equipment may be used much more efficiently when resuscitation is performed by two persons.

Individuals should gain expertise in the use of the equipment mentioned by practising on manikins under the supervision of an instructor.

*Figure 38. Use of a bag/valve/mask unit*

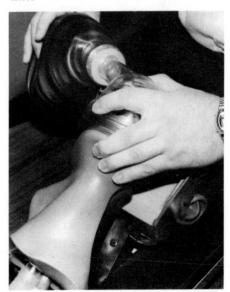

# Tertiary measures

Tertiary measures include improved airway care using the technique of *endotracheal intubation* and the changes this causes to the method of ventilation. The use of the ECG monitor and the diagnosis of the cardiac dysrhythmias present, and the use of the *defibrillator* in the management of ventricular fibrillation are also described.

Also summarised are some of the drugs and intravenous fluids commonly used in the management of cardiac arrest.

## Endotracheal intubation

This is the passing of a *portex* or rubber tube through the vocal cords into the trachea. For the child past puberty and the adult, the tube has a cuff thus preventing the passage of foreign material (e.g. blood or vomit) around the tube into the trachea (Figure 39).

Beside the equipment already mentioned, the following will be required to intubate the patient:
- Endotracheal tube of the appropriate size (see Appendix 3, page 76)
- Laryngoscope (that works!)
- Magill intubating forceps
- 10 ml syringe and artery forceps
- Connection to fit the tube to the bag/valve unit
- Tape to secure the tube to the face
- Stethoscope.

The technique of endotracheal intubation should be taught by a person proficient to do so and should be practised on manikins and anaesthetised subjects. It should *not* be attempted by someone not proficient or trained in the technique. (Further details of the technique will be found in Appendix 3, page 66).

Following endotracheal intubation the tube should be attached to the bag/valve unit, the cuff should be inflated with air from a syringe and the pilot tube clamped off with a pair of artery forceps. The amount of air required to inflate the cuff should be the minimum required to prevent a

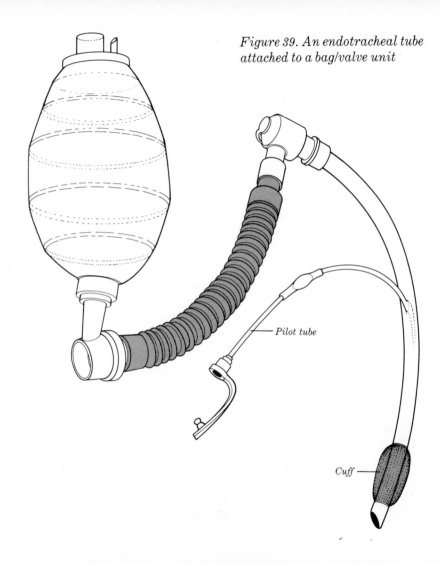

*Figure 39. An endotracheal tube attached to a bag/valve unit*

Pilot tube

Cuff

leak from around it and can best be assessed by blowing up the cuff while the patient is being inflated with the bag and listening for the escape of air from around the cuff. Stop once the escape of air stops.

Also the air sounds should be checked in the apices of both lungs by auscultation with a stethoscope to ensure that the endotracheal tube has not been placed in too far thus only inflating one lung (usually the right lung (Figure 2b, page 4)). One should also ensure that the endotracheal tube has not been inserted into the oesophagus (gurgling is often heard at the end of the tube). The tube should be firmly secured on the outside with adhesive tape to the patient's face (Figure 67, page 73) or with a bandage around the neck, to prevent inadvertent removal of the tube during resuscitation techniques.

With the endotracheal tube in position it is no longer necessary to extend the patient's airway to maintain it. But care must be taken to ensure that the tube is not kinked by the weight of the bag/valve unit if the operator relaxes his hold on it. Also to minimise the risk of the patient biting on the tube during recovery an oropharyngeal airway may be placed in position.

Once the patient is being ventilated with a bag/valve unit attached to the endotracheal tube there is no longer a risk of the air entering the stomach and causing regurgitation of the stomach contents. Any blood/vomit that enters the oropharynx will be unable to pass the cuff on the endotracheal tube and therefore contaminate the airway.

At this stage the airway is absolutely secure, the patient is being ventilated with a bag/valve unit with added oxygen and external chest compression is continuing. Thus our patient should be receiving an oxygenated supply of blood to his brain and other vital organs.

# Diagnosis of type of cardiac arrest

Initially the diagnosis of cardiac arrest has been made and the appropriate signs treated by instituting cardiopulmonary resuscitation.

Now it is important to diagnose the type, and possibly cause, of the arrest and to treat appropriately, reverting the rhythm of the heart to a more normal one. This should also mean the return of a near-normal cardiac output and therefore the end of the cardiac arrest.

The cause of the cardiac arrest may be obvious, e.g. electrocution, drowning, severe blood loss, etc. or may be arrived at by logical guesswork e.g. following myocardial infarction.

*Figure 40. Physio Control Lifepack 5*

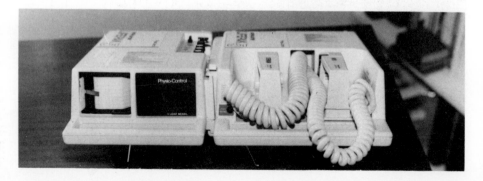

The type of cardiac arrest falls into 3 broad categories:
(1) Ventricular fibrillation.
(2) Asystole.
(3) Electromechanical dissociation.

To be able to assess the type of cardiac dysrhythmia present, firstly we need to connect the patient to an electrocardiograph (ECG) monitor. Depending upon the equipment brought to the patient this may be either a separate monitor or combined with a defibrillator. The equipment may be mains operated, but ideally equipment used specifically in the management of cardiac arrest should be battery operated (Figure 40).

If a combined unit, the ECG may be assessed quickly by simply placing the defibrillator paddles on the patient's chest and observing the ECG on the screen (Figure 41). Otherwise the standard monitoring electrodes may be placed on the patient's chest.

As an alternative, if it is difficult to gain access to the patient's chest because of other personnel involved in the resuscitation, clips or stick-on electrodes may be applied to the patient's wrists (on the inner aspect, which is usually virtually hair-free).

Using a three-lead system:

*Red* – must be on the right side of the heart, i.e. on the upper right side of the chest or on the right arm.

*Yellow* – must be on the left side of the heart, i.e. on the upper left side of the chest or on the left arm.

*Black* – in theory is placed toward the legs, but in practice may be placed almost anywhere. It is often placed on the lower left side of the chest or upper abdomen, but may also be placed on either arm alongside either the red or the yellow. However, the further the black lead is separated from the other two leads the better the ECG trace is likely to be (Figure 42). (If the monitor used gives the choice of leads I, II, or III then it is important that the black lead is below the level of the heart. Otherwise it will only be possible to obtain lead I.)

Once the patient is connected to the ECG monitor it will be necessary to stop ECC to allow recognition of the dysrhythmia as the compression may cause some artefact on the ECG

*Figure 41. Paddle position for 'quick look' ECG monitoring or defibrillation*

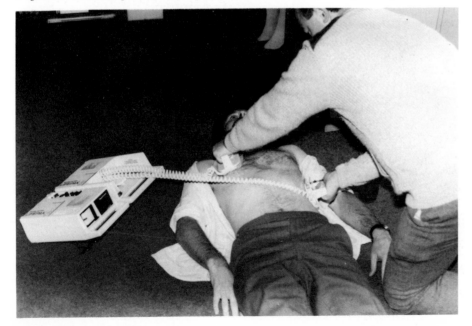

monitor. This delay should not exceed 10–15 sec before ECC is recommended. On recognition of the ECG rhythm the appropriate treatment to revert the rhythm can be commenced. Some ECG monitors have a 'print-out' facility to aid ECG recognition (Figure 40, page 38).

Ventricular fibrillation will require treatment using a defibrillator, whilst asystole and electromechanical dissociation will require appropriate drug therapy (see the following sections).

(See also Appendix 6, page 89.)

# Defibrillation

The idea of using an electric shock in the management of cardiac arrest is not new. The first internal defibrillation of an animal occurred in 1933 and of a human in 1947. But on these occasions it meant opening the chest and applying the defibrillator paddles directly to the heart. In the 1950s W.B. Kouwenhoven defibrillated dogs by applying the paddles to the animals' chests. Soon after this the first human was defibrillated externally. Up to this point *alternating current* (AC) had been used to defibrillate, but it was now found that *direct current* (DC) was more effective and produced fewer side effects.

In the 1960s, the modern defibrillator as we know it came into use.

The defibrillator is designed quite simply to supply a short pulse of electric current to the patient's chest via two electrodes or paddles. Some defibrillators are still only mains operated but most modern defibrillators are battery operated

*Figure 42. Standard electrode position for ECG monitoring*

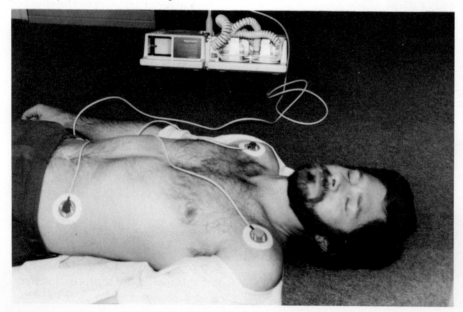

40

(although the batteries are charged via mains or vehicle battery supply). While the defibrillator may take 10–15 sec to charge for use (depending on the level of energy required), the charge when applied to the patient is discharged in a very short time – between 4 and 30 msec.

Normally the defibrillator is used in the management of a fast chaotic ventricular dysrhythmia that results in a total loss of cardiac output – *ventricular fibrillation* (page 106). The energy applied to the heart results in a large mass of the myocardium depolarising at the same time and thus, it is hoped, a more normal rhythm is allowed to 'surface' and control the heart, resulting in a return of cardiac output. If the energy level is not high enough the heart may remain in ventricular fibrillation. If the energy level is too high, the myocardium may be further damaged and/or the rhythm may revert to asystole. However, since time is of the essence, many cardiologists use the highest energy level which they consider to be safe, rather than start at a lower level and gradually increase the energy if the first shock is ineffective.

The amount of energy stored by the defibrillator and delivered to the patient is measured in joules, J (this used to be called watt-seconds). Unfortunately defibrillators are not 100% efficient and deliver less energy to the patient than is stored. Only a few years ago most defibrillators were labelled with the number of joules *stored* by the defibrillator and led one to believe that the same amount was delivered to the patient. Now most defibrillators are labelled with the number of joules actually *delivered* to the patient.

Most modern defibrillators are approximately 80% efficient and therefore when labelled as 100 J stored only actually deliver 80 J, etc. (Figure 43). When only delivered

*Figure 43. Efficiency of defibrillators*

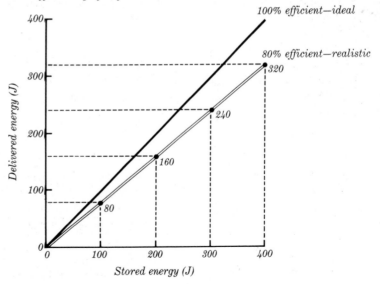

41

energy is indicated on the defibrillator, this has usually taken into account the level of efficiency of energy going through the skin and therefore should be a fairly accurate assessment of the number of joules actually delivered to the heart.

Resistance to the flow of an electric current produces heat. To ensure the minimum amount of resistance as the current passes through the chest wall, it is necessary to use a form of conductive gel between the defibrillator paddles and the chest wall.

Often a gel is spread over the paddles, or some is placed on the centre of a paddle and both paddles are then rubbed together. Unfortunately this is not without its dangers:

(1) Gel may be left on the operator's hands and/or may run along the side of the paddles and come into contact with the operator's hands carrying the risk of the operator receiving a shock when the defibrillator is discharged.
(2) With multiple defibrillation attempts the gel may be spread over the chest wall carrying the risk of the current 'arcing' across the chest wall causing burns.
(3) With use the gel will disappear from the paddles carrying the risk of burns to the patient. Therefore the gel must be replaced/'topped up' between each defibrillation attempt.
(4) If the paddles are placed in the wrong place, gel may be left on the front of the patient's chest, e.g. the sternum. If ECC is attempted the gel may cause the operator to slip, therefore ECC is inefficient.

An alternative which reduces all of these risks is to use electrode gel pads (e.g. 'Defib-pads'). These are squares of electrode gel which are larger than the defibrillator paddles and are placed on the patient's chest where the paddles will be placed. One pad is placed on the upper right side of the chest and the other is placed on the lower left, below the apex of the heart. The paddles can then be placed on the pads without having to have gel placed on them (Figure 44). The defibrillator can be discharged through these pads a number of times without replacing them (they are only used for that one patient). If they become dried at the edges they should be replaced before further defibrillation attempts.

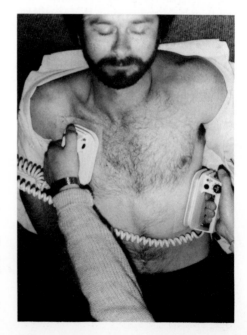

*Figure 44. Paddle position, over Defib-pads, for defibrillation*

The average adult is normally defibrillated at approximately 180–200 J delivered and the amount is increased in increments through to the maximum of 320–360 J (depending upon equipment used) if necessary. For a small adult, the operator may start with 80–100 J (page 87).

When a defibrillator is used it is vitally important that the operator is skilled in its use. This will ensure the safety of the operator and the other personnel. Prior to the defibrillator being discharged, the operator must ensure that no one is in contact with the patient, or anything metal that the patient is in contact with (or is standing in some spilt saline, etc.). If someone other than the patient receives the discharged energy it may cause their heart to go into ventricular fibrillation. If so, commence resuscitation on them, early defibrillation will most likely be successful.

Most of the modern portable defibrillators now available allow the operator to assess the patient's ECG via the defibrillator paddles (Figure 41, page 39). This reduces the time before the patient can be defibrillated and therefore increases the chance of survival. Many would suggest that if a defibrillator is available without an ECG monitor, the patient should be defibrillated anyway. If the patient is in ventricular fibrillation, the sooner he is defibrillated the better, while if he is in asystole or has electromechanical dissociation it is unlikely to do him harm.

## Synchronised cardioversion

This may be used in the management of the patient with a rapid dysrhythmia that may affect the patient's cardiac output, although not cause its total loss (e.g. ventricular or supraventricular tachycardia). On this occasion the defibrillator and monitor are connected so that the energy is discharged only on the R wave of the patient's ECG. This is to ensure that the energy is not delivered in the area of the T wave which may then result in ventricular fibrillation occurring (i.e. R-on-T phenomenon, page 102).

When the defibrillator is in the synchronised mode it will be noted that an artefact is seen on the R wave on the ECG monitor. When the discharge button is pressed there is a slight delay before the defibrillator discharges on an R wave.

If the patient was still conscious prior to the cardioversion attempt he should receive some form of sedation or anaesthesia. He should also be given oxygen (e.g. 4 litres/min via an MC mask) for several minutes before the sedation or cardioversion. It will also be found that the number of joules required to revert the rhythm will be much less than that required in the management of ventricular fibrillation.

*IMPORTANT*
Because of the dangers of misusing the defibrillator, individuals *must* be trained in its use by a suitably qualified and experienced instructor.

# Intravenous infusion

A route is required for the administration of drugs and for fluid replacement where necessary.

Ideally this should be via a large but easily accessible vein, usually in the region of the antecubital fossa, but in the collapsed patient the external jugular vein may be a better alternative, since:

due to peripheral shutdown, the blood is forced back to the heart; as the heart is no longer beating, the blood dams up in the venae cavae and their tributaries, such as the large veins in the neck and thus the neck veins are distended and easy to cannulate;
it is close to the heart and drugs injected into a cannula in it can be flushed down into the heart.

If the intravenous infusion is not already *in situ* a cannula must be sited without interrupting ventilation and ECC. If fluid replacement is going to be necessary (depending on the cause of arrest) one or more large gauge cannulae will be required. If the cannula is required only for the administration of drugs a smaller cannula may be acceptable. If required for drug administration only the cannula may be kept clear during the resuscitation attempt by the slow infusion of a crystalloid, e.g. 5% dextrose solution.

If the patient was previously hypoxic or if the period of circulatory arrest (with effective cardiopulmonary resuscitation) lasts more than 2–3 min, metabolic acidosis will ensue. This will increase the difficulty of reverting the cardiac dysrhythmia that is present.

It has been usual practice to infuse sodium bicarbonate to revert the acidosis. One needs to be careful of the amount infused as it is possible to make the patient alkalotic which also makes it difficult to revert the cardiac arrest.

Efficient cardiopulmonary resuscitation should help to reverse the respiratory acidosis present.

It is now considered that the sodium bicarbonate should be withheld until the blood gases have been assessed.

When given, the sodium bicarbonate should be administered in 50 mmol doses (50 ml of 8.4%) according to the blood gas results.

Individuals involved in the resuscitation attempt must remember that energetic resuscitation may result in the intravenous cannula becoming dislodged. Therefore one must ensure that the cannula and tubing are adequately secured to the patient so that this risk is minimised.

If there is difficulty experienced in finding a suitable vein for the intravenous infusion, some drugs may be administered via the endotracheal route (if an endotracheal tube has been passed). This route may also be used whilst the intravenous cannula is being sited. The dose may need to be increased and there will need to be an adequate volume of fluid (e.g. 10 ml). Do NOT administer sodium bicarbonate via the endotracheal route.

# Resuscitation drugs

There are a number of drugs commonly used in the management of cardiopulmonary arrest. As already mentioned the drugs are usually given intravenously, but may be given via the endotracheal route.

The intracardiac route should no longer be used as there is a risk of unnecessary trauma to the heart, a risk of pneumothorax and a pause is needed in ECC.

The endotracheal route is safe and effective but not all drugs may be given via this route.

The intravenous route is effective when combined with efficient ECC.

In the management of the cardiopulmonary arrest stress, anxiety and the 'adrenaline surge' tend to affect the operator(s). This may result in some difficulty in drawing up the appropriate drugs (risk of ampoules being broken and needles stuck in fingers etc.). As a safe and efficient alternative the drugs needed may be found in

prepacked syringes that minimise the risks/problems involved (e.g. the IMS Min-i-jet system (Figure 45)).

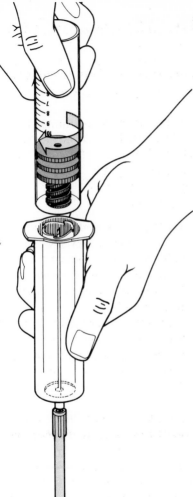

*Figure 45. Min-i-jet system*

On occasion, depending on the mixture of ideas between the individuals present, there may be a great many drugs used during the management of the cardiopulmonary arrest. But those most commonly used at present are:
- Adrenaline
- Atropine
- Lignocaine
- Calcium
- Isoprenaline.

## Adrenaline

Adrenaline is commonly used in the management of asystole and electromechanical dissociation, but may also be used in the management of ventricular fibrillation.

Adrenaline itself has a number of effects on the circulation and these include:

increasing peripheral resistance (without constricting the coronary or cerebral vessels);
raising systolic and diastolic pressure during ECC;
improving, by the above, myocardial and cerebral blood flow;
increasing the contraction of the myocardium;
increasing the irritability of the hypoxic myocardium (i.e. may revert asystole to ventricular fibrillation).

In the management of asystole or electromechanical dissociation, adrenaline may result in the spontaneous return of cardiac action/output. In the management of fine ventricular fibrillation it may coarsen the rhythm and also make the ventricular fibrillation more susceptible to defibrillation attempts.

If adrenaline (10 ml of 1:10 000 solution) is used via the endotracheal route it will improve the coronary blood flow (during ECC) to 25% of pre-arrest level and improve carotid flow even more. Therefore with prolonged cardiopulmonary resuscitation, use of adrenaline increases the chance of change of rhythm to normal and return of cardiac output.

During cardiopulmonary resuscitation 0.5–1.0 mg of adrenaline is given to the patient intravenously (i.e. 5–10 ml of 1:10 000 solution) and can be repeated every 3–5 min as its duration of action is short. This may be given via the endotracheal route in a dose of 1–2 mg in at least 10 ml of volume.

## Atropine

Atropine is used in the management of asystole, giving 2 mg intravenously or 4 mg via the endotracheal route. It is also useful in the management of the patient with an extreme bradycardia resulting in hypotension. Therefore it is probably of more use during the post-arrest phase. It can be of use in the management of atrioventricular block (but not in the management of complete heart block).

It is given intravenously at a dose of 0.5 mg (for an average 70 kg adult) repeated as necessary up to a maximum dose of 2 mg.

## Lignocaine

Lignocaine is still the drug of choice to be used in the management of ventricular dysrhythmias. It will also increase the ventricular fibrillation threshold and therefore is of use in the prevention of ventricular dysrhythmias.

It suppresses myocardial irritability but also causes some myocardial depression, particularly in patients with cardiogenic shock and therefore the amount given may need to be titrated against the effect in these cases.

Lignocaine is used in two strengths, 2% and 20%, and ideally should be used from a prepacked syringe (e.g. Xylocard 2% and 20%).

Initially the 2% is given in a dose of 1 mg/kg body weight intravenously followed by an intravenous infusion of 1g of lignocaine (20% strength) in 500 ml 5% dextrose solution. This should be administered via a burette-type giving set or via an infusion pump supplying 1–4 mg/70 kg per min (1 ml/min will equal 2 mg/min).

If the initial bolus was not sufficient, it may be repeated at a dose of 0.5–1.0 mg/kg every 5 min up to a maximum of 200–300 mg/70 kg.

It must be remembered that lignocaine can cause some central nervous system stimulation (lignocaine 'fit').

Other drugs that may be used include: verapamil, disopyramide, mexiletine, bretylium, procainamide, dopamine, amiodarone, flecainide as well as bronchodilators, diuretics and steroids depending upon the needs of the individual patient.

On recovery appropriate sedation/analgesia may be required along with oxygen therapy.

## Calcium
Calcium is of value during the management of electromechanical dissociation if hypocalcaemia is present, to counteract hypokalaemia or following the use of calcium antagonists. It is usually administered as 10 ml of 10% calcium chloride solution, intravenously, repeated if necessary at 10 min intervals.

## Isoprenaline
Isoprenaline is useful in the management of atropine-resistant bradycardia or very slow, complete heart block prior to pacemaker insertion.

Two mg of isoprenaline (Suscardia) is added to 500 ml of 5% dextrose solution and the flow rate titrated against effect – aim at a ventricular rate of approximately 60–70 b.p.m. (beats per minute). Alternatively dopamine or dobutamine may be infused.

# Effects of cardio-pulmonary resuscitation

Obviously the ideal effect of cardiopulmonary resuscitation is that of survival of the patient and return of normal cardiac, respiratory and neurological function.

The initial basics are aimed at maintaining the viability of the patient and may allow spontaneous recovery. As other techniques are included in the resuscitation attempt it should become a little easier to support the patient and, it is hoped, more likely that recovery occurs. But there may be some problems that occur purely because of the general effect of resuscitation itself upon the patient (or there may be some of the side effects of incorrectly applied cardiopulmonary resuscitation techniques).

With the airway there is little that can go wrong, as long as the airway has been cleared adequately. There is some possibility that extreme backward tilt of the head in the elderly patient with atherosclerosis may lead to some impairment of the vertebral artery–basilar artery system, particularly if the head is also turned to one side. Also some individuals will quote the problems of the fractured cervical spine when discussing airway care. It is possible to maintain the airway without extreme backward tilt and this should be practised on manikins under supervision. This should not, however, discourage individuals from attempting CPR.

When ventilating the patient, hyperventilation (particularly if the patient is a small child) may cause some risk of alveolar damage. But the most probable problem is that of the operator being unable to continue expired air resuscitation because of hyperventilation. Also if the airway is not maintained adequately, it is possible that the air will take the easiest route, i.e. to the stomach, and some regurgitation of the gastric contents may occur with the obvious risk to the airway.

With ECC many individuals are worried about the risk of rib fractures that may occur during 'normal'/correct resuscitation techniques. Some rib fractures may occur, particularly in the elderly patient and this may not be a serious complication. But always ensure that your hand position is correct and your technique is correct (page 20).

If hand position is incorrect, damage to abdominal organs or intrathoracic structures may occur along with the risk of regurgitation of stomach contents with the appropriate risk to the airway.

Probably the greatest problem that occurs during resuscitation attempts is that of the pause – to see what is happening! There should be *no* pause in cardiopulmonary resuscitation of greater than 5–15 sec duration, except to allow for assessment of cardiac output or ECG, to allow for endotracheal intubation, or occasionally intravenous cannulation or movement of the patient. Also, from the safety point of view, one should have a delay in resuscitation to allow for defibrillation but the resuscitation attempts should recommence again after defibrillation. There should not be the usual long delay whilst individuals decide what is on the monitor, etc.

# Successful or?

If the resuscitation attempt is successful, in that the patient's respiratory and circulatory systems are being supported, there will be some improvement in the patient's physical condition.

There should be some improvement in the patient's general colour, the eyelash-reflex may be seen to have returned. If there is no associated cerebral damage the pupils will start to constrict and to react to light. There may be some spontaneous movement by the patient, particularly clenching of the jaw.

As recovery continues the patient may start to make some effort to return to normal respiratory movement. Continue to ventilate the patient, timing your ventilations to coincide with the patient's inspiration, until the patient is breathing adequately for himself (blood gas analysis may be necessary).

There may be the spontaneous return of palpable pulses (carotid or femoral), if so, external chest compression should be discontinued.

Conversely, if after 30–60 min of cardiopulmonary resuscitation none of the above are noted, the patient does not respond to any stimulus, there is no respiratory effort, no palpable pulses and the pupils remain fixed and dilated, the time may have arrived where the continuation of resuscitation needs to be questioned. If the patient is being monitored and any form of dysrhythmia (other than asystole) is noted, resuscitation may need to continue. Also, if there is any likelihood of poisoning and/or hypothermia, resuscitation may need to be continued until death can be established without any doubt.

There will be the occasion where cardiopulmonary resuscitation has been started and very soon after information is received which suggests that resuscitation is inappropriate (e.g. incurable/terminal disease). Or, due to obvious injuries, resuscitation is inappropriate and was not commenced initially (e.g. decapitation). But often resuscitation may have been started and it then becomes difficult to merely abandon the patient.

Normally one would expect that the senior doctor present will be able to decide when resuscitation is no longer appropriate and stop further resuscitation attempts, but on occasion (e.g. in the community) the doctor may not be available – then the rescuer may need to make the decision.

If the rescuer is physically unable to continue the resuscitation attempt the decision has then been made, but more often the rescuer may have reached the 30–60 min stage with no signs of life from the patient and the rescuer has to make the decision to abandon the resuscitation attempt.

# Aftercare

Following successful resuscitation the patient may require artificial ventilation if only the circulatory function has returned. If breathing adequately for himself the airway will still need to be maintained until the patient is fully conscious. Some vomiting may occur during this recovery phase.

The conscious patient will need a great deal of reassurance and may need sedation or analgesia (depending upon the individual needs).

Oxygen therapy may need to be continued (depending upon blood gas analysis) and one should assess the cause of arrest, if known, and try to prevent further occurrence by appropriate prophylactic treatment.

General observation of the patient can be continued along with the assessment for injuries that may have been received during the resuscitation attempt.

The patient may require further management of other medical problems e.g. pulmonary oedema, cerebral oedema, cardiogenic shock, etc.

It may be noticed (particularly by the relatives) that there is some degree of cerebral impairment following the period of arrest. This may improve.

Also, unfortunately, there may be the need for long term care of the patient who physically recovered from the period of arrest but has severe cerebral damage.

The relatives should be allowed/ encouraged to discuss their feelings regarding the physical/mental state of the patient following the cardiac arrest. Depending upon the overall prognosis, other disciplines may be involved in the care of the patient and relatives.

During the aftercare one may need also to look at the support required for individuals who were involved in or who witnessed the resuscitation sequence, particularly junior/inexperienced staff, other patients or relatives. They may be very distressed by the occurrence, especially if the patient died.

# Future developments in cardio-pulmonary resuscitation

New ideas are at present being tried and used, e.g. the administration of adrenaline via the endotracheal tube. Work by N. Chandra, M.T. Rudikoff and M.L. Weisfeldt indicates that ventilation at the same time as ECC will increase the carotid flow. This involves timing ventilation to occur at exactly the same time as ECC, as opposed to the occasional coincidence. But for this, obviously the patient must have an endotracheal tube *in situ*.

Some other work under investigation in Los Angeles concerns the use of pulsation from a pressure suit around the lower part of the body.

But something that does appear to be in use now and could easily be taught is cough CPR.

### Cough CPR

It was found by Dr J.M. Criley in 1976 that individuals in ventricular fibrillation could remain conscious if they coughed, particularly if it was repetitive vigorous coordinated coughing. In the laboratory individuals have been able to remain conscious for $1\frac{1}{2}$ min by this method before being defibrillated.

At present it is not known how long one can maintain an adequate oxygen supply to the brain by this method.

It has been suggested by Dr P. Safar that if a monitored patient develops ventricular fibrillation he should be encouraged to cough until a defibrillator is available. Also that patients at risk of cardiac arrest could be taught, if they feel their heart has stopped, to cough forcibly once a second and take deep breaths between coughs (calling for help and hoping that it will keep them conscious until help arrives).

One should also be aware of the possible risks that forced coughing may have on the patient who has not arrested but does have coronary artery disease. It may cause dysrhythmias or even cardiac arrest or at the least fainting.

# Appendixes

## Appendix 1: Treatment of choking

Many individuals of all ages die every year because of sudden total airway obstruction – choking.

Often witnesses strike the patient on the back, but frequently with no real result. In patients who have been found in a state of cardiac arrest cardiopulmonary resuscitation has been implemented but often with an unsuccessful outcome. All too often the cause of death is to be found wedged in the trachea – the 'café coronary'.

All this led to some work in the early 1970s by Professor H.J. Heimlich in the USA. His results and suggestions were reported in 1974 and by 1975 the 'Heimlich technique' was being taught and saving lives.

When someone is choking they are frequently unable to make any sound (i.e. they have a completely obstructed airway) and are literally minutes from death. If still conscious it will be noticed that the patient often clutches at his throat and may become cyanosed. If asked 'are you choking?' the patient may be able to nod but not speak.

Alternatively the patient may have already collapsed due to hypoxia and is found apparently having had a cardiac arrest. It will then be noted that in spite of apparently clearing the airway and then attempting expired air resuscitation no air enters the lungs. The rescuer may then reattempt to clear the airway and try to ventilate again. If still not successful, assume a total airway obstruction.

So what do we do about it?

### Heimlich technique
If the patient is still conscious and upright, tell the patient what you are going to do and stand behind him. Place your arms around the patient, placing one fist against the patient's upper abdomen above the umbilicus but below the end of the sternum.

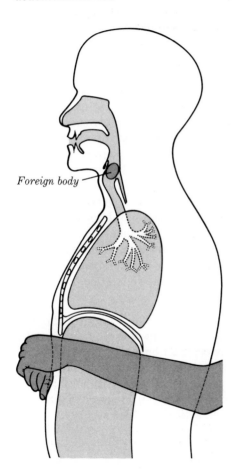

*Figure 46. The hand position for abdominal thrust*

Foreign body

Grasp that fist with your other hand (Figure 46). Thrust your fist into the patient's abdomen with an upward movement (Figure 47) (the direction of movement is in and up toward the diaphragm), sharply and firmly several times. This should result in the movement of the obstruction out of the patient's mouth, or at least into the mouth from where it can be easily removed (Figure 48, page 56).

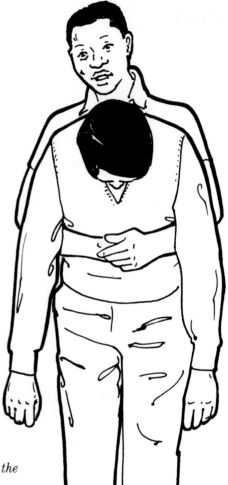

*Figure 47. Abdominal thrust – the upright position*

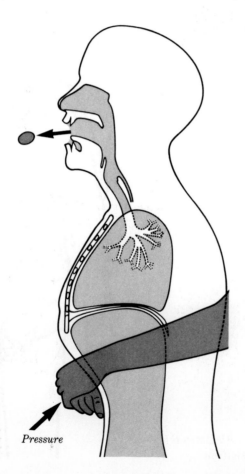

*Figure 48. Removal of an obstruction from the airway*

Pressure

If the patient is too large for you to manage to encircle the abdomen, encourage the patient to lie down. Or if the patient has lost consciousness and is on the ground, place the patient on his back with the head facing up (turning the head twists the airway and may prevent the obstruction from being removed – if the patient vomits, clear the airway and then continue). Straddle the patient's legs with yourself facing up the patient's body toward the head. Place your hands as if you were going to commence ECC but with the heel of your hand on the abdomen between the umbilicus and the lower end of the sternum. Give a sharp, firm thrust in and up toward the diaphragm and repeat several times (Figure 49).

This should result in movement of the obstruction out of the airway. Usually the obstruction is actually ejected from the mouth, but if not, sweep your fingers around the mouth, making sure you do not push the obstruction back down.

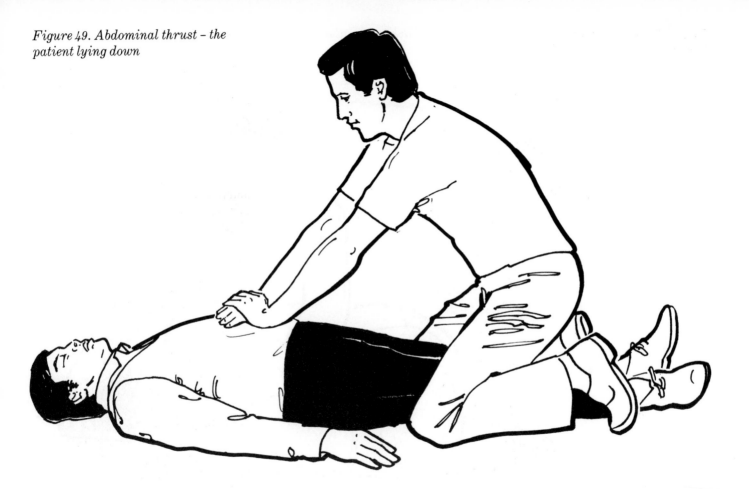

*Figure 49. Abdominal thrust – the patient lying down*

If the Heimlich technique is unsuccessful, it may be worthwhile turning the patient onto his side and striking the back (between the shoulder blades) with the heel of your hand (Figure 50) and then repeating the Heimlich technique.

*Figure 50. Back blow – adult*

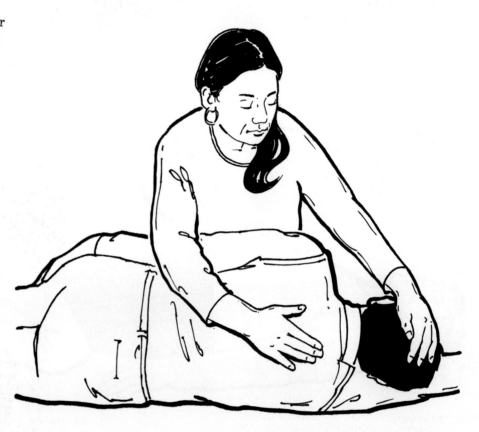

If the patient is still upright, back blows may be administered in this position (Figure 51). (Some individuals do not believe that back blows are very effective.)

Continue until successful. Implement resuscitation if the patient remains in a state of cardiac arrest after the obstruction has been cleared.

As an alternative in the very obese individual or in the pregnant female when there is no room between the top of the uterus and the chest, chest thrusts may be used.

Continue as with the Heimlich technique but place your fist/hand on the centre of the sternum. This method carries a high risk of rib fractures and related trauma. Therefore always use the Heimlich technique/abdominal thrust in preference (even with pregnant females the abdominal thrust can be used safely as long as there is a space between the top of the uterus and the lower end of the sternum).

In the infant, the Heimlich technique can still be used (although some recommend that only chest thrusts

*Figure 51. Back blow – upright position*

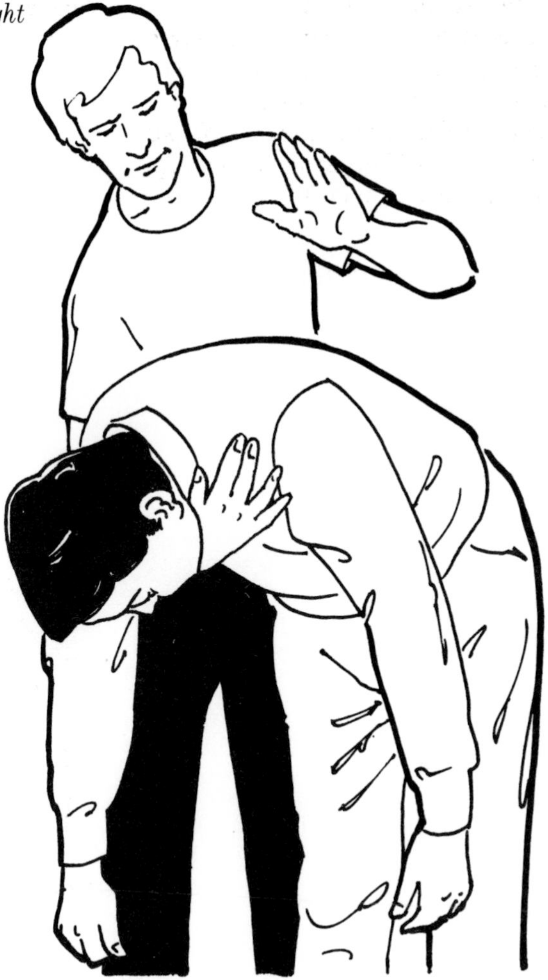

are used because of the risk of damage to the liver with abdominal thrusts), but use only the index and middle fingers of each hand with the child on your lap (Figure 52) or on its back on a firm surface.

*Figure 52. Chest thrust – Infant*

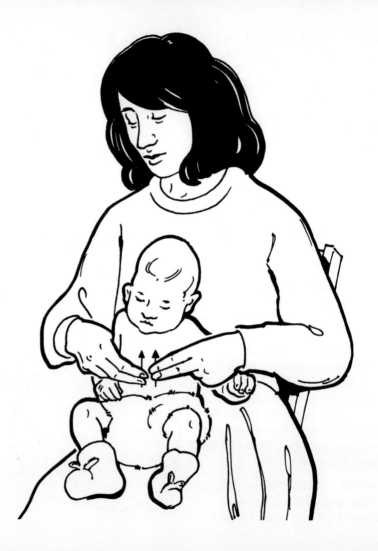

If repeated attempts with this technique fail an alternative is to place the infant/child over your arm/thigh with the head dependent and strike between the shoulder blades with your other hand or hold the child by the ankles (head down) and strike him between the shoulder blades (Figures 53 and 54, page 62).

*Figure 53. Back blow – infant*

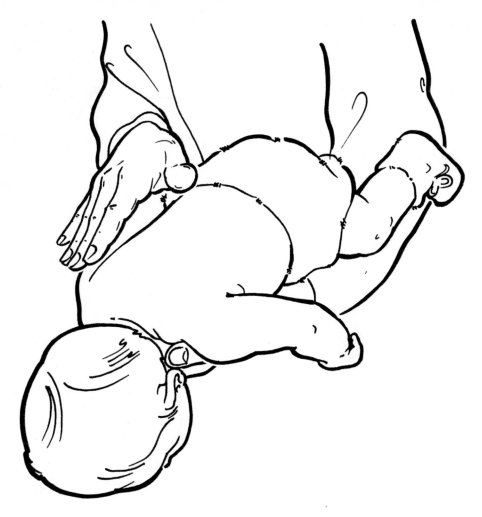

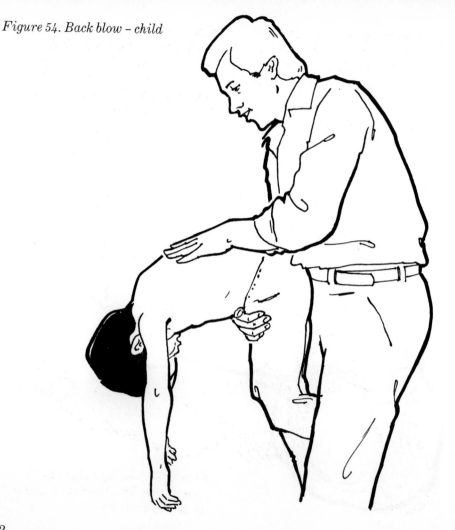

*Figure 54. Back blow – child*

This method is dangerous and may result in trauma if too much force is used or the obstruction may fall forward and lodge against the vocal cords. Therefore, if possible, use the Heimlich technique.

The other advantage of the Heimlich technique is that if it is you who is choking and you are alone or no one else helps, you may be able to clear the obstruction yourself by lying against the top of the back of a wooden chair and dropping your weight on to it, so that the top of the chair is forced into your abdomen between umbilicus and sternum in an upward direction toward the diaphragm.

# Appendix 2: Recovery position

If an unconscious patient is left on his back the airway may become obstructed by the tongue or contaminated by regurgitated gastric contents.

Obviously if the patient requires expired air resuscitation or external chest compression then the patient needs to be left on his back – but if the patient is breathing and sustaining an adequate circulation, the airway is the priority.

If the unconscious patient is placed on his/her side the tongue tends to fall forward and any gastric contents, or blood, saliva etc. that may contaminate the airway, can drain out.

The position the patient is placed in has had a number of names over the years and at present is known as the *recovery position*.

There are a number of minor variations in the way the patient is turned and positioned, all having the same overall effect. The actual technique used may vary with the needs of the individual patient, the amount of space available and the expertise of the operator.

The operator must kneel at one side of the patient. The patient will be turned toward the operator on every occasion. Do not roll the patient away from yourself as you will have no control over the patient's movement.

Place the patient's arm that is nearest to you up alongside the patient's head and cross the leg farthest from you over the one nearest to you (Figure 55(a)). Place the other arm across the patient's chest/abdomen.

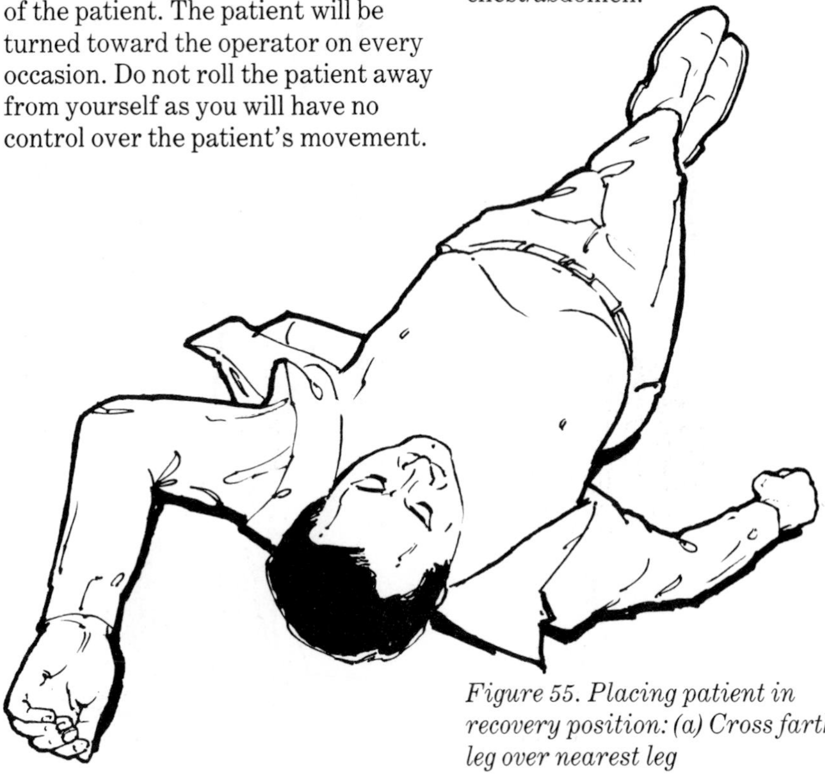

*Figure 55. Placing patient in recovery position: (a) Cross farthest leg over nearest leg*

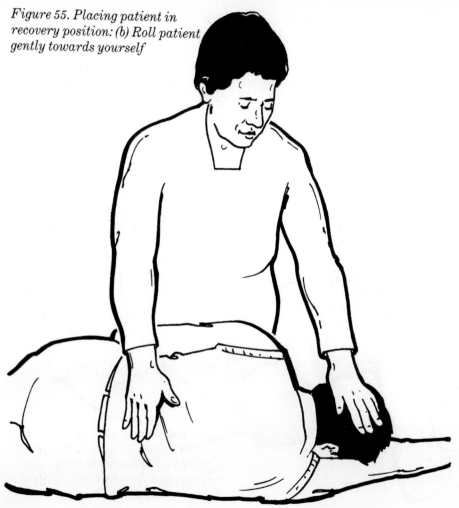

*Figure 55. Placing patient in recovery position: (b) Roll patient gently towards yourself*

Then grasp the patient's shoulder and hip farthest from you (it may be easier to grasp the clothing) and, using your own weight, pull the patient toward you.

It will be found that the patient's head will rest on his outstretched arm and that will have prevented the head from hitting the floor. The other arm can now be used to support the upper part of the body by resting it against the ground and the leg that was bent can be brought up further toward you to support the lower part of the body (Figure 55(c)).

The patient will remain comfortably in this position without further support from yourself. The only disadvantage of using this technique is that the arm the head is resting on extends beyond the head. This may be in the way if the patient is placed on a stretcher.

64

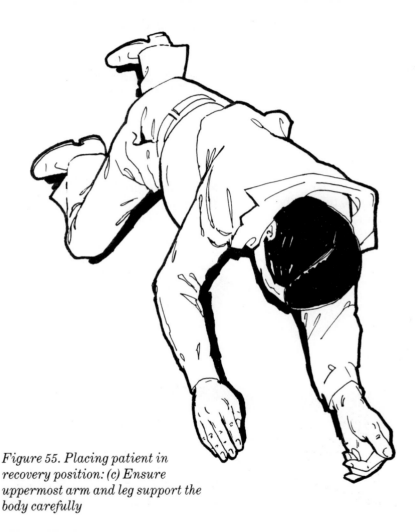

*Figure 55. Placing patient in recovery position: (c) Ensure uppermost arm and leg support the body carefully*

An alternative method is to place the arm nearest yourself under the patient's side, cross the other arm across the chest/abdomen and pull up the leg nearest to you (i.e. bend it at the knee and pull the heel toward the buttocks). Pull the patient toward you but ensure that the head is protected as otherwise it will strike the ground. Once the patient is over, place the hand of the arm now nearest you under the head to support it. Ensure the body is off the other arm by pulling it out behind the patient.

With both methods, ensure that at the end of moving the patient, the airway is still clear, the head is extended sufficiently and the patient is breathing adequately.

(There is another variation that is taught by some organisations but it does not support the head and it is felt by the author that one or other of the above will be adequate.)

65

# Appendix 3: Endotracheal intubation

Endotracheal intubation is the passing of a plastic or rubber tube into the trachea so that its end is past the level of the vocal cords. In patients over about 12 years the tube used has a cuff on it which is inflated distal to the vocal cords to prevent foreign material entering the airway around the tube.

Endotracheal intubation is probably the safest way of maintaining the airway in a deeply unconscious patient. But its use is not without some dangers. This section is merely to give some theoretical insight into the technique and to explain the equipment needed.

The technique of endotracheal intubation itself should be taught by a person proficient to do so and practised on manikins and/or anaesthetised subjects. It should NOT be attempted by someone not proficient or trained in the technique.

## Equipment

Besides the airway, suction and ventilation equipment mentioned under the primary and secondary measures the following are also required:

- a laryngoscope (Figure 56) (an instrument with a light source that is used to enable the operator to view the vocal cords);
- an endotracheal tube of the appropriate size (plus one larger and one smaller size) (see table, page 76);
- a pair of Magill forceps (may be necessary to guide the endotracheal tube into place);
- 10 ml syringe and artery forceps (if using a cuffed tube);
- a connection to fit the endotracheal tube to the bag/valve unit;
- tape to secure the tube in place;
- stethoscope (to check air entry at both lung apices after intubation).

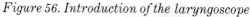

*Figure 56. Introduction of the laryngoscope*

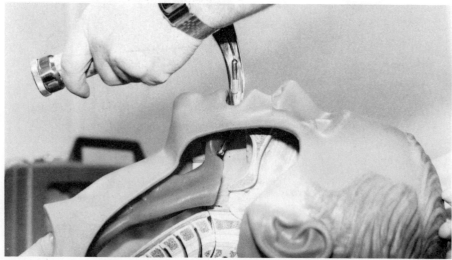

## Technique

When performing endotracheal intubation ensure all the equipment required is at hand.

With the non-breathing patient, he must be adequately ventilated first and the technique should take as little time as possible. If some difficulty is encountered in the intubation attempt causing a delay, then the attempt should be stopped and the patient ventilated with a bag/valve/mask unit to ensure adequate oxygenation before the next attempt.

One of the major problems that arises during the attempted intubation of a patient following cardiac arrest is that of the operator failing (or refusing) to recognise the difficulties being encountered and the patient becoming more and more hypoxic while the attempt continues.

It is imperative that there is a minimal delay/pause in the ventilation of the non-breathing patient (intubation should not take longer than 10–15 sec).

The technique itself, in theory, is straightforward. Place yourself behind the patient's head facing down the length of the body. The head is placed in the 'sniffing the morning air' position: flexing the cervical spine by putting the patient's head on a pillow, then extending the head on the top of the spine (atlanto-occipital joint) (Figure 57). This is to ensure as straight a line as possible between the line of the oropharynx and the line of the trachea; the neck is *not* hyperextended (Figure 58). It may help to place something (e.g. a small pillow) under the patient's head, but not near the shoulders. If the head is correctly positioned in the first place, many of the difficulties encountered can be eliminated.

The laryngoscope is a left-handed instrument and is therefore held in the left hand throughout the procedure and not swapped from hand to hand.

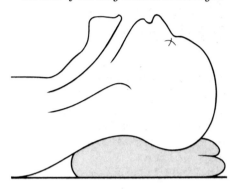

*Figure 57. 'Sniffing the morning air' – the line of airway should be straight*

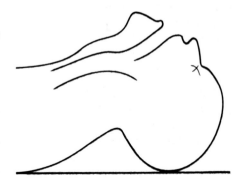

*Figure 58.* Incorrect *position for endotracheal intubation – the neck is extended; the line of airway curved*

It is introduced into the right side of
the mouth and gently moved into the
mid-line therefore pushing the tongue
to the left (Figure 59).

*Figure 59. The laryngoscope blade
slides over the tongue*

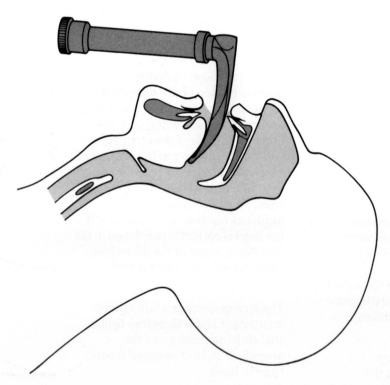

The handle of the laryngoscope is lifted in the direction in which it points. The operator must resist the temptation to pull back on the handle as this then results in the laryngoscope using the patient's upper jaw/teeth as a fulcrum resulting in trauma to the upper teeth (Figure 60).

*Figure 60. Lift the laryngoscope in the direction of the handle*

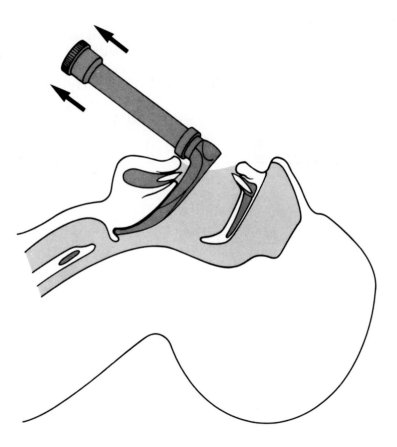

The operator must also ensure that the patient's lip is not caught between the laryngoscope blade and the teeth (Figure 61).

*Figure 61. The danger of catching a lip between the laryngoscope blade and teeth*

If a laryngoscope with a curved blade is used the tip of the blade is advanced and slides into the vallecula (the angle between the base of the tongue and the epiglottis). If a laryngoscope with a straight blade is used the tip of the blade is placed posterior to the epiglottis and is used to pull the epiglottis anteriorly. At this point the laryngeal opening should be in view. If there is still some difficulty in viewing the vocal cords, gentle pressure on the larynx by an assistant may make the procedure easier (Figure 62).

*Figure 62. A view of the vocal cords*

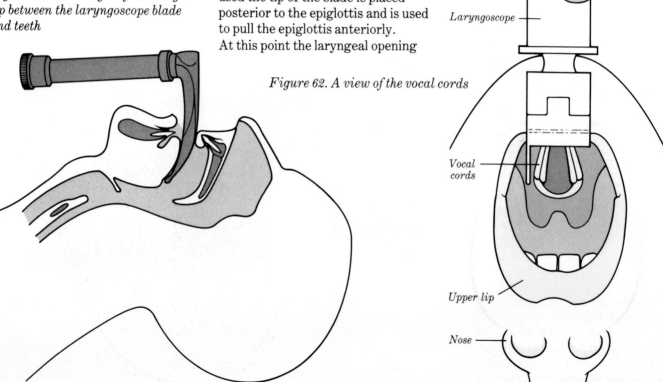

Laryngoscope

Vocal cords

Upper lip

Nose

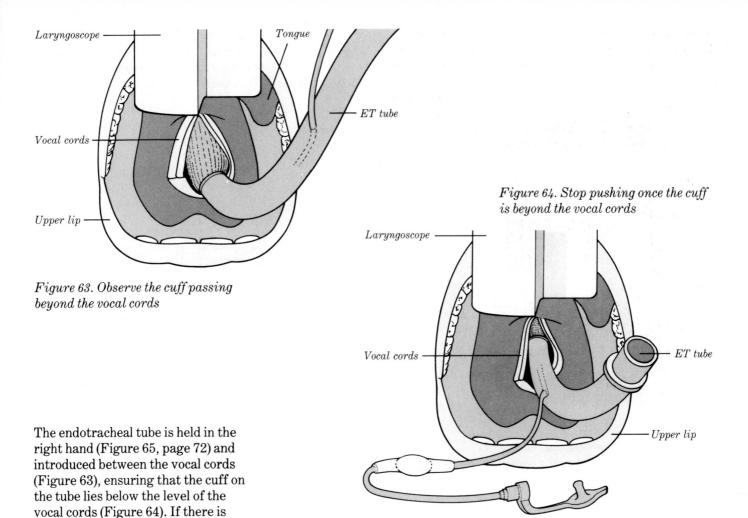

Laryngoscope

Tongue

ET tube

Vocal cords

Upper lip

*Figure 63. Observe the cuff passing beyond the vocal cords*

*Figure 64. Stop pushing once the cuff is beyond the vocal cords*

Laryngoscope

Vocal cords

ET tube

Upper lip

The endotracheal tube is held in the right hand (Figure 65, page 72) and introduced between the vocal cords (Figure 63), ensuring that the cuff on the tube lies below the level of the vocal cords (Figure 64). If there is

71

*Figure 65. Holding the laryngoscope with the left hand, introduce the endotracheal tube with the right*

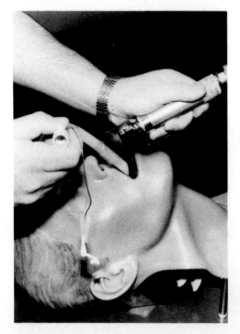

some difficulty in passing the endotracheal tube through the cords, the procedure may be helped by the use of the Magill forceps or an introducer in the endotracheal tube.

Once the endotracheal tube is in position the laryngoscope can be removed. A bag/valve unit can be attached to the endotracheal tube and ventilation of the patient recommenced. The cuff on the endotracheal tube is inflated sufficiently to prevent a loss of air from around the cuff (Figure 66).

*Figure 66. The cuff of the endotracheal tube inflated below the cords – safeguarding the airway*

The operator must listen for breath sounds at the apex of each lung to ensure that the endotracheal tube is correctly positioned.

A common problem is for the endotracheal tube to be pushed too far, allowing it to enter the right main bronchus, and therefore the left lung may not be ventilated. If this

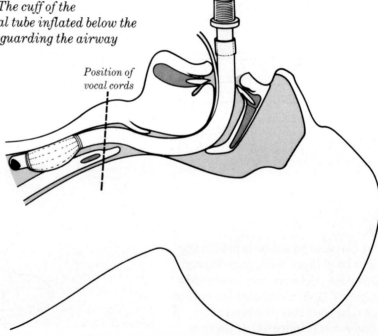

Position of vocal cords

occurs, *deflate* the cuff and pull the tube back slightly and recheck. Then reinflate the cuff.

Once the tube is in the correct position secure the endotracheal tube to the patient with adhesive strapping or bandage (Figure 67).

*Figure 67. Ensure that the endotracheal tube is secured in position to prevent inadvertent removal*

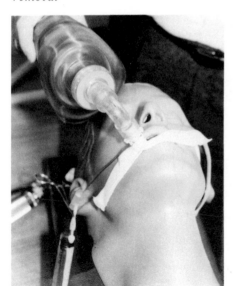

It may well be wise to also place an oropharyngeal airway in position. As the patient's level of consciousness improves the airway will prevent the patient from 'clamping' his teeth on the endotracheal tube.

*Figure 68. The laryngoscope may be used to aid airway care in combination with the suction booster*

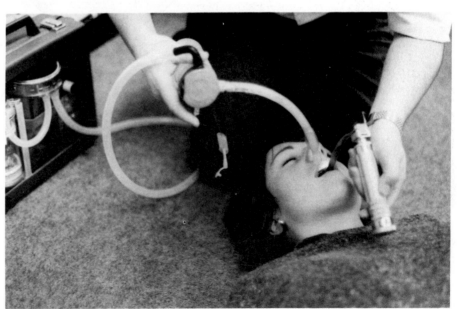

The laryngoscope may also be used as an aid to airway care. It will allow the operator to gain a much better view of the oropharynx when removing foreign material with Magill forceps or suction equipment (Figure 68, below and Figure 69, page 74).

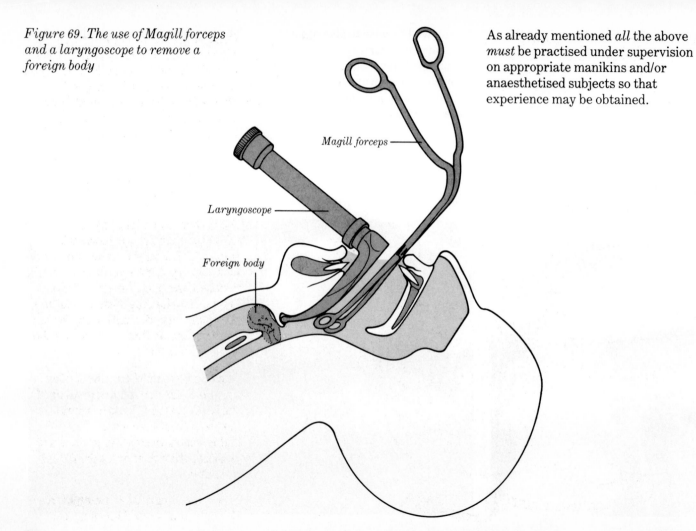

*Figure 69. The use of Magill forceps and a laryngoscope to remove a foreign body*

Magill forceps

Laryngoscope

Foreign body

As already mentioned *all* the above *must* be practised under supervision on appropriate manikins and/or anaesthetised subjects so that experience may be obtained.

A number of problems may arise because of anatomical differences etc., and each of these should be explained by, and discussed with your instructor in the practical setting (Figure 70).

*Figure 70. The danger of the tube entering the oesophagus*

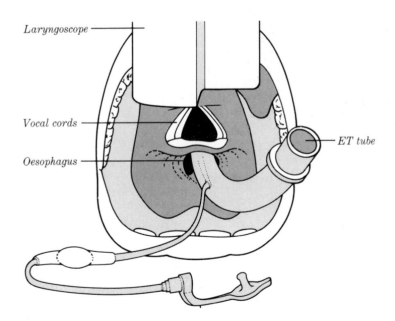

Laryngoscope

Vocal cords

Oesophagus

ET tube

**Oesophageal obturator airway**
This is a cuffed tube (very much like an endotracheal tube) that is attached to a face mask. The lower end is blocked and there are a number of small holes in the part of the tube that will lie in the oropharynx.

The single sized tube may be inserted into the oesophagus of deeply unconscious individuals. The aim is to occlude the oesophagus totally, once the cuff has been inflated, and prevent regurgitation of gastric contents. The tube does *not* ensure a patent airway, the operator must still maintain the backward tilt of the head. With the face mask in position the patient can be ventilated, the air entering the patient's airway via the holes in the tube.

The oesophageal obturator airway may be of use in the management of the cardiac arrest if there are no personnel experienced in endotracheal intubation but it is *not* an alternative to endotracheal intubation.

It has the advantage of being of one size only and is relatively easy to insert. There is some risk of damage to the oesophagus and the risk of inadvertent tracheal intubation and asphyxia (which should not be a problem if immediately recognised).

Its use is contraindicated in patients who have swallowed caustic substances, patients who are known to have oesophageal disease and anyone under the age of 16 years.

A modified oesophageal obturator airway is the oesophageal gastric tube airway. This uses the tube itself for gastric drainage and has no holes at the pharyngeal level. Ventilation is via a separate port on the mask, the same as using a bag and mask.

Removal of the airway may be followed by regurgitation of stomach contents; therefore ensure the recovering patient has a cough reflex before removing the airway. If the patient is still unconscious, the mask may be disconnected and an endotracheal tube passed before the airway is removed. Efficient suction equipment is obviously required.

## Sizes of endotracheal tubes

The size (internal diameter) of the endotracheal tube may be established by dividing the age of the patient by 4 and adding 4.5. Because of the variation in the size of the larynx of individuals of the same age it is usual to have one larger and one smaller tube as well.

*Range of sizes*

| Age | Weight (kg) | Internal diameter (mm) | Approximate length of tube (cm) | |
|---|---|---|---|---|
| | | | Oral | Nasal |
| Premature | 1.0–2.0 | 2.5 | 8 | 9 |
| Newborn | 2.0–2.5 | | | |
| 0–3 months | 2.5–5.0 | 3.5 | 10 | 12 |
| 3–6 months | 5.0–9.0 | 4.0 | 11 | 14 |
| 6–12 months | | 4.5 | 12 | 15.5 |
| 1–2 years | 9.0–11.0 | | | |
| 2–4 years | 11.0–16.0 | 5.0 | 13 | 17 |
| 4–5 years | 16.0–20.0 | 5.5 | 14 | 18.5 |
| 5–7 years | | 6.0 | 15 | 20 |
| 7–8 years | | 6.5 | 16 | 21 |
| 8–10 years | | 7.0 | 17 | 22.5 |
| 10–12 years | | 7.5 | 18 | 24 |
| 12–14 years | | 8.0 | 19 | 25 |
| Adult female | | 8.0–9.0 | 20–26 | 26–29 |
| Adult male | | 8.5–10.0 | 22–28 | 26–32 |

The length of the tube for oral intubation may be assessed by measuring the distance from the lobe of the ear to the angle of the mouth and doubling it.

For emergency use the tube may be cut approximately to size beforehand. Usually this means that the tube will be slightly long. It is important in this case to check that the tube has not been placed in the right main bronchus, and that if the position is correct in the trachea that the tube outside the mouth is not allowed to kink over (with the weight of the bag/valve/unit) and therefore occlude the airway.

# Appendix 4: Hypothermia

Every year many people, particularly the young and the elderly, suffer the effects of hypothermia. At one end of the scale, it may merely result in discomfort or confusion but at the other may lead to death.

Let us consider what hypothermia is, the effects it has on the patient and why this is of importance when considering cardiac arrest and resuscitation.

By definition hypothermia is:
<u>a dangerous lowering of the body temperature.</u>
This means that the patient has a rectal or oesophageal temperature of less than 35°C (95°F). We must ignore skin temperature as there may be some considerable difference between the temperature of exposed skin and that of the body's core. In fact blood supply to the skin will have been reduced to try to maintain heat in the core.

Normally as our body is affected by the cold we react voluntarily by clothing ourselves appropriately, and/or involuntarily, by reducing the blood supply to the skin (minimising heat loss) and initiating shivering (creating heat). The very young may be unable to clothe themselves, the elderly may be less aware of the fact that they are getting cold (due to lack of proper regulatory control) and any individuals may be affected by poor housing/heating/food intake or the effect of drugs that may reduce the awareness of the individual to the cold or even abolish shivering, e.g. various sedatives and alcohol. An acute medical emergency or trauma (e.g. 'collapse', unconsciousness, injuries preventing movement etc.) may have resulted in the individual becoming totally unable to react to the fact that they are getting cold. As the individual becomes hypothermic they become less aware of their surroundings, they progressively lose consciousness and breathing and cardiac output gradually deteriorate. The patient's skin will obviously feel cold, but more important, the skin that should be warm is cold, e.g. skin on the abdomen that is normally covered by clothing.

If the temperature is to be assessed accurately a suitable low-reading thermometer or probe should be inserted into the rectum, or a suitable probe inserted into the oesophagus. In the pre-hospital setting, the core temperature should not be measured if it entails removal of clothing in a hostile environment. The level of hypothermia may be assessed by looking at the patient's responses/reactions and clinical observations, then applying them to the following chart.

The hypothermic individual who is breathing and who has a pulse may be rewarmed by preventing further heat loss:

- wrap in a 'space blanket' and add blankets;
- gradual (passive) rewarming by nursing in a warmed room (23–30°C), aiming at a rise of core temperature of approximately 0.5°C per hour;
- in the pre-hospital phase of patient management, depending upon circumstances, the above may be used or a more active form of reheating – that of the *buddy treatment*. Place the patient in a sleeping bag, having removed any wet clothing and place another warm individual in the sleeping bag with the patient.

If the patient is found cold but conscious do NOT encourage exercise as a method of rewarming. It may be found that the blood in the periphery (limbs) may be much colder than the core and by encouraging physical activity in the patient the colder blood may be 'dumped' in the core. This may result in a rapid drop in the core temperature which may then be sufficient to cause circulatory collapse.

At this point we must remember that the individual who is found very hypothermic, e.g. with a core temperature of 30°C, may appear very cold and totally unresponsive to any stimuli, may have rigid muscles, no tendon reflexes, dilated pupils and, most important, a respiratory effort so slow and shallow it may not be obvious and a pulse so weak it may not be felt. Over the years a

*Table of signs related to core temperature*

| Signs | Core temperature (°C) |
|---|---|
| Shivering. | 35–36 |
| Confusion and disorientation. | 34–35 |
| Amnesia. | 33–34 |
| Cardiac dysrhythmias, shivering replaced by muscle rigidity. | 33 |
| Progressive loss of consciousness until the patient is totally unresponsive. Pupils dilate; loss of tendon reflexes. | 30–33 |
| Ventricular fibrillation may occur. | 28 |

significant number of patients over the country have been thought to be dead and have 'woken up' in the mortuary!

We must also remember that the patient who is profoundly hypothermic and has had a cardiorespiratory arrest may survive the period of hypoxia/anoxia for a longer period of time than the non-hypothermic arrest. This is because the hyopthermic patient's metabolic rate is greatly reduced: there are a number of individuals on record who have survived apparent death with a total recovery (including no neurological deficit).

Therefore, whether the patient is hypothermic and appears to have had a cardiorespiratory arrest or is found in a state of cardiorespiratory arrest and appears to be hypothermic, resuscitation should be implemented to maintain an adequate oxygenated circulation within the body. The problem then is that the patient may need rewarming before the cardiorespiratory arrest can be reverted. This may take some hours and full resuscitative measures will need to be continued throughout this time.

Probably the best way to warm this patient is to ventilate him with warmed/humidified gases (oxygen) and therefore warm the core of the body. This may be attempted using a soda lime canister in circuit with a manual resuscitator (in the pre-hospital setting) but is probably best accomplished by using a heated humidifier on a mechanical ventilator.

Attempts should continue until either the patient's core temperature rises and it is possible to revert the dysrhythmia etc., or the patient's core temperature rises and it becomes obvious that resuscitation attempts are no longer warranted, or a decision to abandon resuscitation is made by a suitably experienced senior doctor.

If the patient is profoundly hypothermic do not be in a hurry to abandon resuscitation, particularly if the patient is a child. The heart and nervous system of children have an extraordinary resistance to hypoxic damage.

# Appendix 5: Paediatric resuscitation

The basic principles of management of cardiorespiratory arrest in the child follow the teachings of resuscitation for adults, but there are some fairly important differences related to differences in the anatomy and physiology of the child compared with the adult. The following adjustments then need to be made to the techniques of resuscitation.

In this appendix I do not intend to discuss resuscitation of the newborn. The practical aspects of resuscitation of infants and children should be practised under the supervision of a suitably qualified instructor, using paediatric manikins.

For the purposes of cardiorespiratory resuscitation, I am defining an infant as being under 12 months of age and a child as being between 1 and 8 years of age. A child over 8 years of age may be managed as an adult.

I intend to cover each of the steps already mentioned in adult resuscitation and mention the appropriate differences. It should be remembered that children who suffer cardiorespiratory arrest usually only have one main problem and prognosis is usually good (unlike the adult with coronary artery disease, etc.). Also often the cause of arrest in the child is hypoxia and respiratory arrest, it is not usually of cardiac origin. Therefore, once hypoxia is relieved, management of the arrest may be successful.

**Airway**

In the non-breathing infant/child the airway must be assessed and cleared. There may be some foreign body occluding the airway, e.g. vomit, milk, food in the infant, sweets, toys, etc. in the child. This may be removed by a finger sweep or back blows with the child/infant in the head-down position. Abdominal thrusts are not recommended in infants and children because of the risk of damage to the abdominal organs, but chest thrusts may be successful.

Once the airway is clear it will need to be maintained by tilting the head back – do NOT hyperextend the neck in the infant/child as this may result in occlusion of the airway by the softer structures of the neck (Figure 71). Oropharyngeal airways may be used with great care as it is very easy to cause trauma to the airway and if the airway is being successfully maintained without an oropharyngeal airway *in situ* it may be better not to insert one.

*Figure 71. The correct position for airway improvement – do not hyperextend the infant's neck*

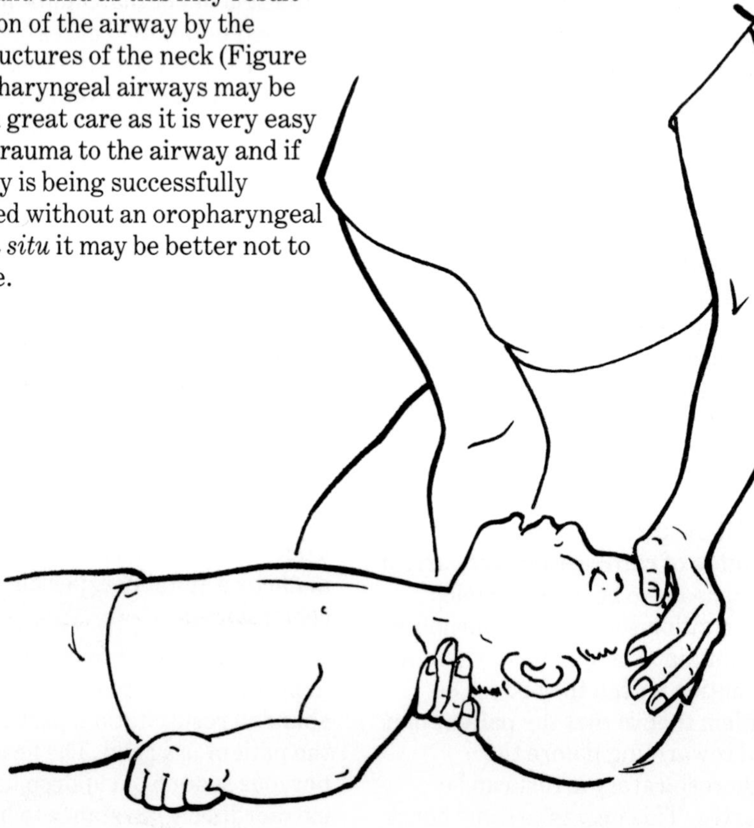

In the majority of occasions the airway can be maintained by simple means and endotracheal intubation is not required. If it is required, it should only be performed by someone experienced and competent in this technique with children and infants.

**Breathing**
The non-breathing infant/child may be ventilated using EAR (mouth-to-mouth and nose method) (Figure 72).

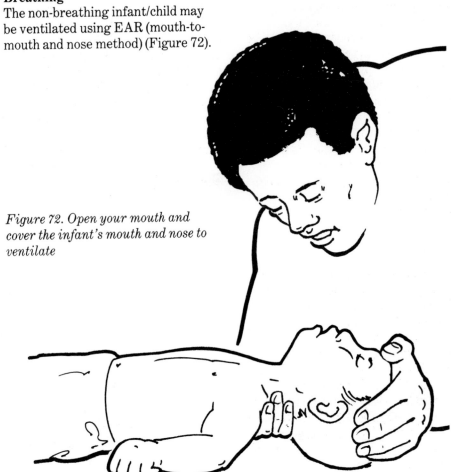

*Figure 72. Open your mouth and cover the infant's mouth and nose to ventilate*

An alternative is to use a
bag/valve/mask unit (Figure 73).

*Figure 73. Infant resuscitation with
two persons*

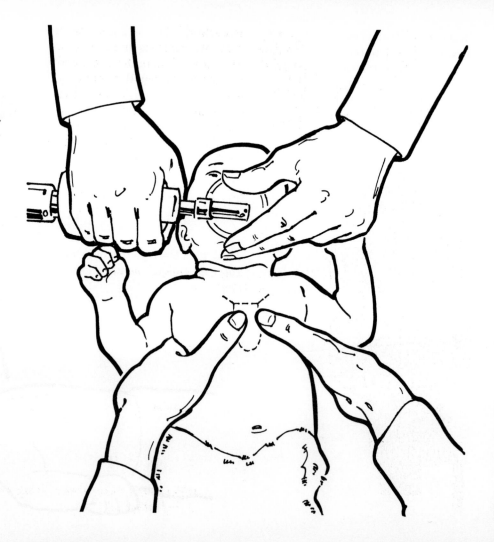

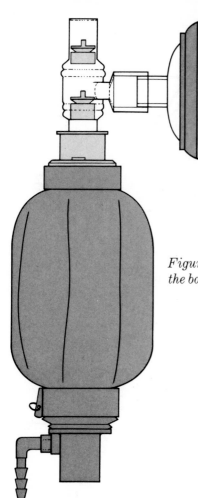

If using EAR in the infant, use only puffs of air from your cheeks (it is easy to overinflate the infant and rupture the lungs). With both methods use only sufficient air to cause the chest to rise. If using a bag/valve/mask unit add oxygen if possible and ventilate if possible with 100% oxygen (Figures 74 and 75).

Ventilate the infant at a rate of 20–30 times per minute and the child at a rate of 15–20 times per minute.

*Figure 74. An Ambu resuscitator – the baby model*

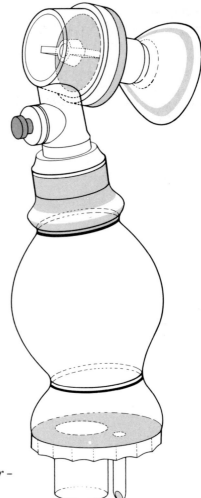

*Figure 75. A Laerdal resuscitator – the infant model*

## Circulation

In the infant it is difficult to feel the carotid pulse because of the short neck, therefore assess the brachial or femoral pulse (Figure 76). In the child assess the carotid, brachial or femoral pulse.

*Figure 76. Feel the brachial artery to assess the heart rate*

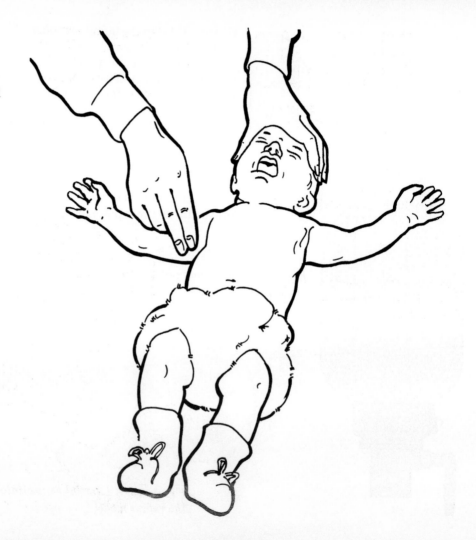

If no pulse initiate ECC. Do NOT attempt to use a precordial thump in infants or children – it is rarely successful and likely to cause trauma.

ECC in the infant may be performed by encircling the chest with both hands and exerting pressure on the mid point of the sternum (the heart is higher in the chest and there is less risk of damaging other organs, e.g. liver) with both thumbs (Figure 77).

*Figure 77. ECC – encircle the infant's chest with your hands and compress with the thumbs*

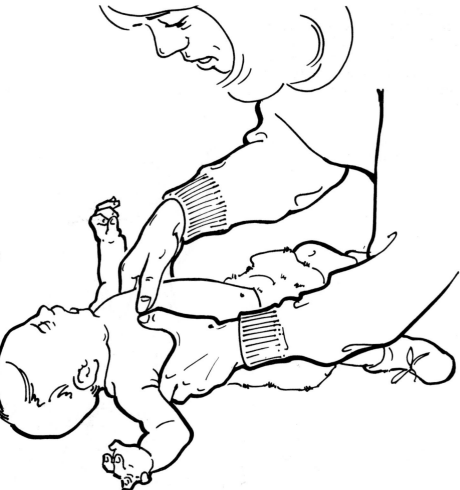

Alternatively, use two fingers of one hand on the mid sternum but ensure that the infant is on a firm surface (Figure 78). It will be noted that there is a gap behind the infant's back and if ECC is to be effective this gap must be filled. It is often easiest to do this with one hand whilst performing ECC with the other. The rate of compression in the infant is 100 per minute with a depth of depression of $\frac{1}{2}$–1 in (1.5–2.5 cm).

*Figure 78. Press two fingers on the infant's sternum*

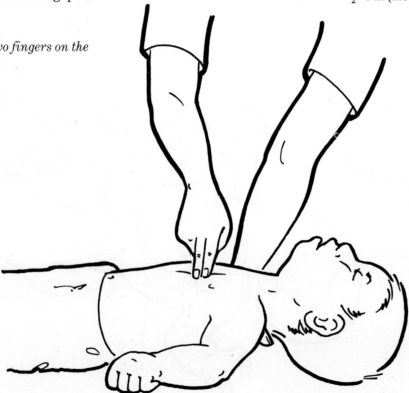

In the child ECC is performed using the heel of one hand on the mid sternum compressing at a rate of 80/min with a depth of depression of 1–1½ in (2.5–3.0 cm) (Figure 79).

Continue ECC with a smooth action and not sharp jerks.

If combining EAR with ECC, continue at a rate of one breath to five compressions with one or two operators.

**Diagnosis** – ECG
The ECG monitor, when available, may be connected to the child as for the adult. It may often be found that the infant/child, because of hypoxia causing the arrest, is in an extreme bradycardia or asystole. Ventricular fibrillation may, however, be the result of electrocution, electrolyte imbalance or the effect of drugs.

**Defibrillation**
If in ventricular fibrillation or ventricular tachycardia with no cardiac output the infant or child may be defibrillated. It is important that the appropriate size paddles should

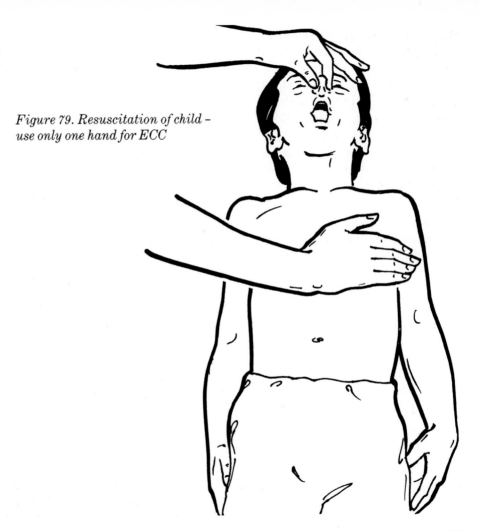

*Figure 79. Resuscitation of child – use only one hand for ECC*

be fitted to the equipment (4.5 cm in diameter for infants and 8 cm diameter for children).

The infant/child is defibrillated at a level of 2 J/kg, and if that is not successful it may be increased to 4 J/kg. If this is still unsuccessful appropriate drug therapy should be started.

**Drugs**
The same drugs used in the resuscitation of adults will be used but in a different dose.

There may also be some difficulty in actually gaining access to a suitable vein to allow the administration of drugs. It may be necessary to delay intravenous cannulation until the experienced paediatrician is available. Some drugs may be given via the endotracheal route if the patient is intubated.

It will be necessary to treat the acidosis that will have occurred. Ideally arterial blood gas results should be obtained and the administration of sodium bicarbonate must depend upon those results.

Sodium bicarbonate solution must always be given intravenously. If the needle or cannula slips out of the vein inadvertently, and the solution is given into the tissues, necrosis of the tissues may follow.

*Drugs commonly used in the management of cardiac arrest*

| Drug | Dosage | Reason for administration |
|------|--------|---------------------------|
| Adrenaline 1:10 000 solution | 0.1 ml/kg | Asystole, extreme bradycardia, fine ventricular fibrillation |
| Calcium chloride 10% | 0.1 ml/kg | Electromechanical dissociation |
| Lignocaine 2% | 1 mg/kg | Ventricular dysrhythmias |
| Atropine 0.5 mg/ml | 0.01 mg/kg | Sinus bradycardia |
| Isoprenaline 2 mg/2 ml | By infusion – add 2 mg to 500 ml 5% dextrose (gives 4 $\mu$g/ml); administer at a rate of 0.1–0.5 $\mu$g kg/min | Extreme bradycardia, complete heart block, poor cardiac output. |

Some drugs may be given via the intracardiac route, but, as mentioned previously, this will result in a delay/pause in ECC and may result in laceration of the myocardium.

It should be remembered that hypoglycaemia is often associated with cardiorespiratory arrest in infants and therefore 1 ml/kg body weight of a 50% dextrose solution may be worth administering to the patient.

Dopamine may be of use post-arrest if there is still a poor cardiac output.

# Appendix 6: ECG recognition

For a full understanding of cardiac dysrhythmias the student should refer to a suitable text on the recognition of dysrhythmias† along with discussion of simulated dysrhythmias on a cardiac dysrhythmia simulator with a suitably qualified instructor.

Generally when assessing the ECG the observer must always relate the ECG monitor to the patient. If there appears to be an abnormality on the ECG monitor but the patient is conscious, alert and not distressed in any way, there is no need to rush over and worry the patient. There may merely be a problem with the leads or monitor. Alternatively, one can observe a 'normal' ECG on the monitor and the patient may have had a cardiorespiratory arrest, because of electromechanical

†For example, J. Gardiner, *The ECG – What does it tell?* (Stanley Thornes (Publishers) Ltd, 1983).

dissociation (electrically the heart is functioning, mechanically it is not).

The observer must be able to recognise the rhythm that is normal for that patient, i.e. a rhythm that results in a normal cardiac output that is adequate for that individual and that is not likely to cause any serious or life-threatening dysrhythmia.

These rhythms could include: sinus rhythm, bradycardia, tachycardia or arrhythmia, first-degree heart block, occasional atrial ectopics, atrial flutter or fibrillation, junctional rhythm (of a rate to maintain an adequate cardiac output).

Next the observer must be able to recognise the rhythms that may cause some reduction in cardiac output, often by first noting the effect on the patient, i.e. dizziness etc. These may include a very slow sinus bradycardia or junctional rhythm, a very fast sinus tachycardia, a fast atrial dysrhythmia, supraventricular tachycardia.

The observer must be able to assess warning dysrhythmias i.e. those that may well lead to a life threatening dysrhythmia: second-degree heart block (particularly mobitz type 2), ventricular ectopics (particularly if multifocal), R-on-T ventricular ectopics, ventricular tachycardia.

Finally, obviously the observer must be able to recognise the rhythms that either result in such a gross reduction of cardiac output that it is potentially life threatening or actually result in a total loss of cardiac output and therefore in cardiac arrest. They include: complete heart block, ventricular tachycardia, ventricular flutter and fibrillation, ventricular standstill, asystole.

The following sections are taken from J. Gardiner, *The ECG – What does it tell?*

# Sinus rhythm

## Description

Normal rhythm, with the impulse originating in the sinoatrial node, and following a normal pathway (Figure 80).

## ECG characteristic

■ Rate: 60–100 b.p.m.

■ Rhythm: regular

■ P waves: normal, preceding each QRS complex

■ P–R interval: normal (0.16–0.2 sec)

■ QRS complex: normal

## Clinical significance

Nil, as this is a normal rhythm, therefore no treatment is required.

*Figure 80. Sinus Rhythm*

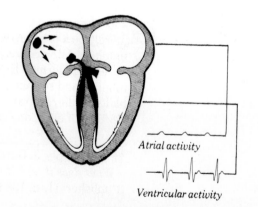

*Atrial activity*

*Ventricular activity*

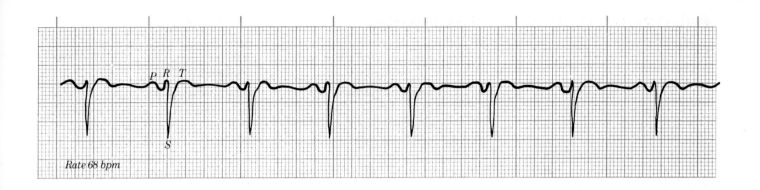

P R T

S

Rate 68 bpm

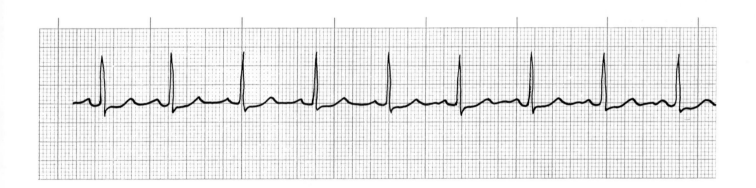

# Sinus bradycardia

## Description
Impulse originates in the sinoatrial node (Figure 81).

## ECG characteristic
- Rate: below 60 b.p.m. (usually 40–60)
- Rhythm: regular
- P waves: normal
- P–R interval: normal
- QRS complex: normal

## Clinical significance
May be normal in athletic young adults, or due to increased parasympathetic tone (vagus nerve), damage to S–A node, hypoxia or excess of cardiac drugs (such as *digoxin, propranolol*).

The slow rate may result in a lowering of the blood pressure and deterioration in tissue perfusion.

## Treatment
No treatment is required if the blood pressure is maintained and the patient is unaffected generally.

However, treatment may be required if:

(1) Blood pressure is unduly lowered (systolic < 100 mm Hg).
(2) Skin is pale, cold and clammy.
(3) There is agitation, confusion, dizziness or unconsciousness.
(4) Ventricular dysrhythmias appear.

The drug of choice is *atropine sulphate* (600 μg (0.6 mg) in 1 ml) in a dose of 0.6–1.2 mg i.v. to increase the heart rate.

The patient should also be placed flat to assist cerebral supply, and oxygen therapy given to reduce the risk of cerebral hypoxia (which may be causing the bradycardia).

*Figure 81. Sinus bradycardia*

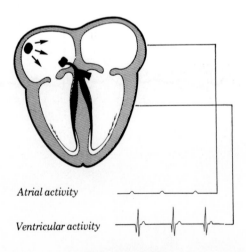

Atrial activity

Ventricular activity

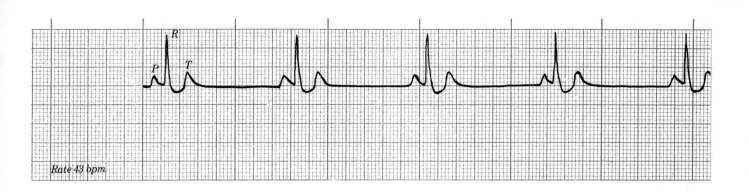

P R T

Rate 43 bpm

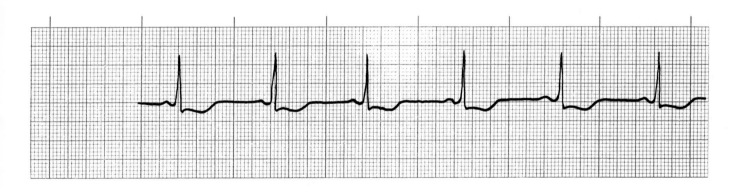

93

# Sinus tachycardia

## Description
Impulse originates in the sinoatrial node (Figure 82).

## ECG characteristic
- Rate: 100–180 b.p.m.
- Rhythm: regular
- P waves: normal; if the rate is very fast the P wave may be buried in the T wave of the previous beat
- P–R interval: normal
- QRS complex normal

## Clinical significance
May be due to increased sympathetic stimulation caused by pain, fever or anxiety, or may be the normal reaction to exercise. It may also be due to haemorrhage, early hypoxia, congestive cardiac failure, left ventricular failure, or overdose of drugs such as *atropine, adrenaline, isoprenaline* or *aminophylline*.

If the rate is not too high there may be little effect on the patient. If over 120–140 b.p.m. the cardiac output may be reduced due to decreased ventricular filling time. This may result in a lowered blood pressure, reduced tissue perfusion and its associated signs and symptoms.

The increased cardiac workload, but decreased coronary supply to the myocardium, may result in myocardial ischaemia and the possibility of chest pain.

## Treatment
Relieve pain if present by *entonox* or other analgesia; reassure the patient: relieve anxiety (with *Valium* if necessary); relieve hypoxia with oxygen therapy; control haemorrhage; treat heart failure, if present, by *digoxin* and diuretics.

*Figure 82. Sinus tachycardia*

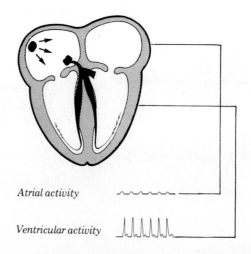

Atrial activity

Ventricular activity

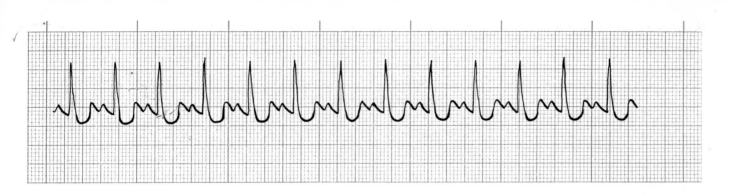

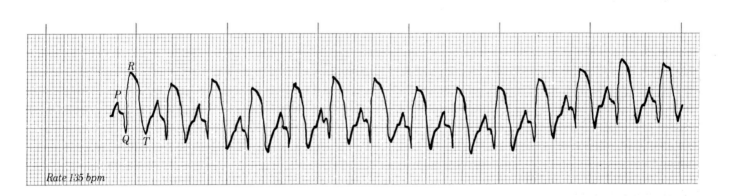

Rate 135 bpm

95

# Premature atrial contractions (atrial ectopics)

## Description

A premature beat arises from an ectopic focus which originates an impulse before the next normal beat is due. Therefore in an otherwise 'normal' rhythm an ectopic beat appears. The R–R interval between the ectopic beat and the previous normal beat will be less than the normal R–R interval. The R–R interval between the ectopic beat and the following normal beat may be longer than the normal R–R interval. The pause after the ectopic beat, and before the next normal beat, is known as a *compensatory pause*. After the atrial ectopic the rhythm returns to normal until the next ectopic beat (Figure 83).

## ECG characteristic

- Rate: normal
- Rhythm: basically regular except for the atrial ectopics

- P waves: basically normal, but abnormal prior to the atrial ectopics

- P–R interval: normal, except that of the atrial ectopic and then will vary depending upon the site of the ectopic focus.

- QRS complex: normal

## Clinical significance

Premature atrial contractions may be a normal phenomenon and may be caused by emotional disturbances or the use of tobacco, tea or coffee. They may also be due to digoxin toxicity or to organic heart disease causing damage to the atrial wall. The presence of atrial ectopics (if very frequent) may be a warning of other atrial dysrhythmias.

## Treatment

Usually no treatment required unless:

(1) The dysrhythmia is due to digoxin toxicity, assess blood level and alter the regime.

(2) The dysrhythmia is due to atrial damage/heart failure, in which case digoxin or β-blockers may be prescribed.

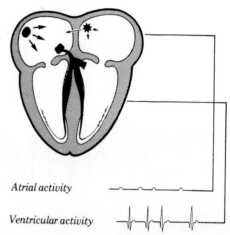

*Figure 83. Premature atrial contractions*

*Atrial activity*

*Ventricular activity*

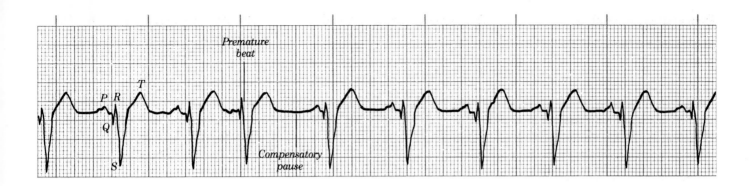

Premature beat

P R T

Q

S

Compensatory pause

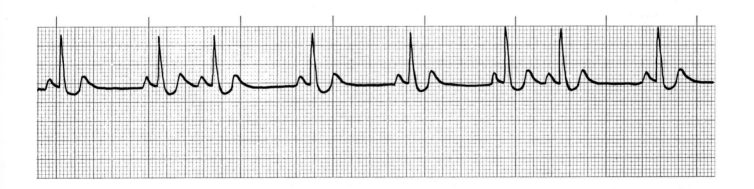

# Supraventricular tachycardia

## Description
The impulses originate from somewhere within the atria (including the S–A node and A–V node). Because of the rapid ventricular rate (>150/min) P waves cannot be identified so neither can the exact origin of the impulse. This term is therefore used as a blanket term when the rhythm originates above the ventricles (supraventricular) and because of the rapid rate it is difficult or impossible to identify the rhythm accurately (Figure 84).

The arrhythmia may appear as paroxysms which start and end suddenly.

## ECG characteristic
■ Rate: 160–210/min (can reach 300/min in infants)
■ Rhythm: regular
■ P waves: cannot be identified
■ P–R interval: cannot be identified
■ QRS complex: normal, but occasionally an abnormality in the conduction of the impulse down the bundle branches (bundle branch block) may widen the QRS complex and it may then be difficult to differentiate between supraventricular tachycardia and ventricular tachycardia.

## Clinical significance
May occur for no apparent reason or may be due to damage to the S–A node, atria or A–V node (because of ischaemic heart disease). May also be caused by drug excess or sympathetic overactivity.

The very rapid rate will result in a lowering of cardiac output, with accompanying hypotension, poor tissue perfusion and cerebral hypoxia. The patient may complain of chest pain because the rapid rate may result in some myocardial ischaemia.

## Treatment
Oxygen therapy or entonox may be required to treat the hypoxia and/or chest pain. Reflex vagal stimulation can be used (for example, carotid sinus massage or supraorbital pressure), in conjunction with monitoring of ECG and pulse, to reduce the rate; verapamil (Cordilox) 5 mg i.v. may be used (can be repeated, if necessary), or $\beta$-blockers (such as *practolol* (10 mg in 5 ml), 5–20 mg i.v. slowly (at approx. 1 mg/min)) have been successful in treating the dysrhythmia.

If unsuccessful other drugs such as digoxin or similar may be used, or elective cardioversion (especially if the cardiac output is very low).

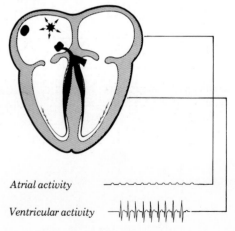

*Figure 84. Supraventricular tachycardia*

*Atrial activity*

*Ventricular activity*

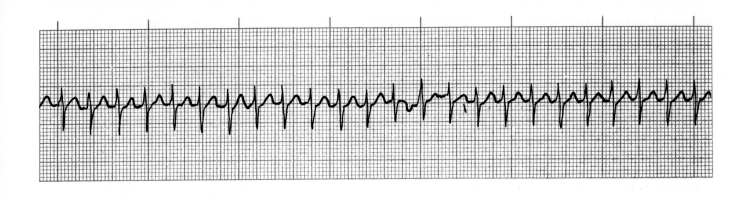

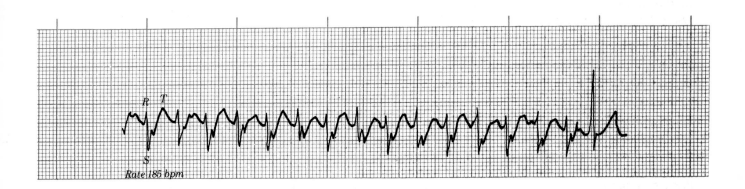

Rate 185 bpm

# Premature ventricular contractions (ventricular ectopics)

## Description
The impulse originates somewhere within the ventricular myocardium. It is a premature beat arriving before the next normal beat is due and is followed by a compensatory pause. The QRS complex is wide and bizarre-looking (greater than 0.12 sec in duration) and the T wave is usually in the opposite direction to the QRS complex. The ectopic beat may just appear singly in an otherwise normal rhythm (Figure 85).

## ECG characteristic
- Rate: normal
- Rhythm: regular except for ventricular ectopics
- P waves: not seen
- P-R interval: not identifiable
- QRS complex: wide and bizarre (greater than 0.12 sec – three small squares).

## Clinical significance
May be caused by damage to the ventricles (ischaemic heart disease), increased sympathetic or parasympathetic activity, hypoxia, acidosis, congestive cardiac failure or an overdose of some drugs.

Isolated ventricular ectopics may not be significant, but more frequent ventricular ectopics may result in a slight reduction in cardiac output, or may be the precursor of more serious ventricular dysrhythmias.

## Treatment
May solely be observation (if the ectopics are associated with ischaemic heart disease), but if the ventricular ectopics are very frequent and/or lead to a lowering in cardiac output treat with *lignocaine* (see ventricular tachycardia, page 104).

*Figure 85. Premature ventricular contraction*

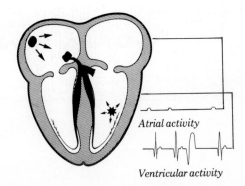

*Atrial activity*

*Ventricular activity*

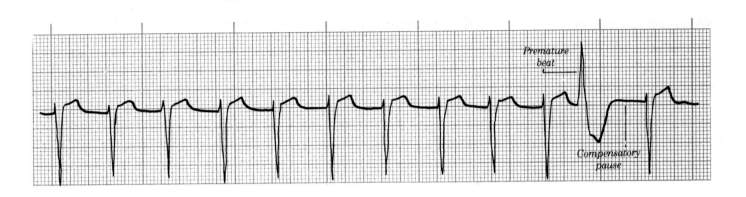

*Premature beat*

*Compensatory pause*

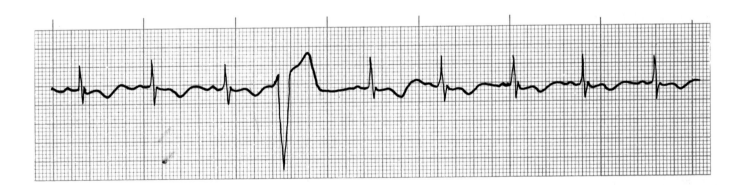

101

# R-on-T ectopics

## Description
The impulse originates somewhere in the ventricular myocardium, the same as ventricular ectopics (VEs). But with this type of VE the impulse is initiated earlier still so that the R wave of the VE lands on the T wave of the previous beat (in other words depolarisation starts to occur while repolarisation is still occurring) (Figure 86)

## ECG characteristic
- Rate: normal
- Rhythm: regular, except for the VEs
- P waves: not seen
- P–R interval: not identifiable
- QRS complex: wide and bizarre (greater than 0.12 sec), with the R wave of the VE apparently running off the T wave of the previous beat.

## Clinical significance
The same as for VEs but with a greater risk of more serious ventricular dysrhythmias. Because depolarisation starts again while repolarisation is still occurring there is an increased risk of ventricular fibrillation.

*Figure 86. R-on-T ectopic*

## Treatment
Close observation and drug therapy (lignocaine i.v.) as soon as possible (see ventricular tachycardia, page 104).

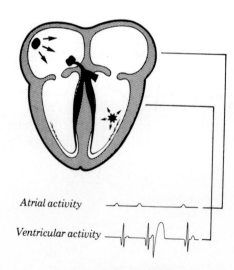

Atrial activity

Ventricular activity

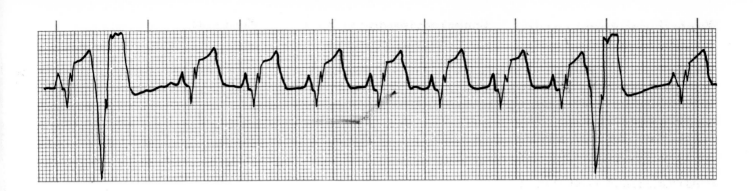

103

# Ventricular tachycardia

## Description

Impulses originate from somewhere within the ventricular myocardium, appearing as three or more ventricular ectopics in a row. The ectopic foci may fire off at a rate of 140–220 b.p.m. It may sometimes be difficult to distinguish between ventricular tachycardia and supraventricular tacycardia, but note that ventricular tachycardia is slightly irregular while supraventricular tachycardia is regular (Figure 87).

## ECG characteristic

- Rate: usually 140–220 b.p.m.
- Rhythm: slightly irregular
- P waves: usually present but may be buried in the QRS complex
- P–R interval: unidentifiable; the atria and ventricles are dissociated from each other
- QRS complex: wide and bizarre (greater than 0.12 sec)

## Clinical significance

The rhythm may be caused by damage to the conduction pathway or ventricles (ischaemic heart disease), increased sympathetic or parasympathetic tone, hypoxia, acidosis, low serum potassium or overdose of some drugs.

If the rate is over 120–140 b.p.m. the cardiac output may be significantly affected resulting in a drop in both tissue perfusion and blood pressure. The signs and symptoms noted would be those of poor tissue perfusion and hypotension, and the rapid heart rate may be associated with myocardial ischaemia (angina) and pump failure. The dysrhythmia itself can be extremely dangerous resulting in unconsciousness and even death. Ventricular tachycardia may be a precursor of ventricular fibrillation.

## Treatment

If the patient is conscious, lignocaine is the drug of choice, given as: 2% lignocaine (100 mg in a prepacked 5 ml syringe) at a dose of 1 mg/kg body weight i.v. (50–100 mg i.v. in the average adult). The dose may be repeated once more if necessary.

Care must be taken when giving lignocaine i.v. because if given too quickly it may cause cerebral irritation resulting in a 'lignocaine fit'.

The i.v. dose should be followed by an intravenous infusion of 5% *dextrose with lignocaine* (5 ml of 20% lignocaine = 1000 mg, is added to 500 ml of 5% dextrose and run through a Metriset at 60 drops/min (60 ml/hour)).

If the patient loses consciousness because of an inadequate cardiac output, observe closely as he may lose his cardiac output completely, in which case treat as cardiac arrest.

Other antiarrhythmic drugs can be used such as mexiletine or disopyramide.

*Figure 87.*

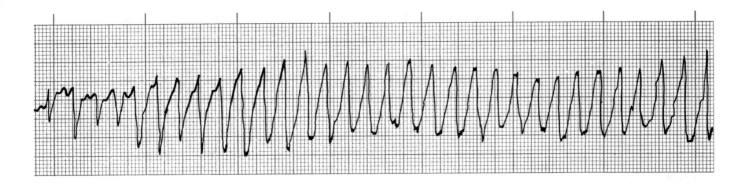

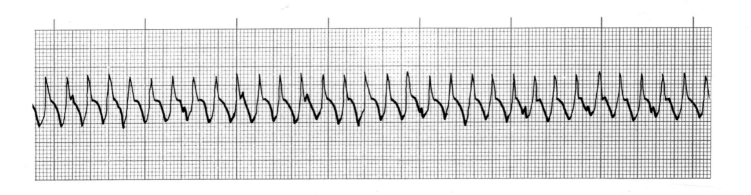

# Ventricular fibrillation

## Description
Impulses originate in one or more foci within the ventricles at a very fast rate, resulting in an uncoordinated activity within the ventricular myocardium (Figure 88).

## ECG characteristic
- Rate: difficult to ascertain, fibrillation waves are seen at a rate in excess of 300/min
- Rhythm: irregular, uncoordinated, chaotic
- P waves: may or may not be present, but anyway are unrecognisable
- P–R interval: absent
- QRS complex: absent. The ectopic foci result in waves of fibrillation of varying amplitude and shape. The waves are known as coarse or fine depending upon amplitude.

## Clinical significance
May have the same causes as the other ventricular dysrhythmias. Ventricular fibrillation will result in a total loss of cardiac output, and cause cardiac arrest.

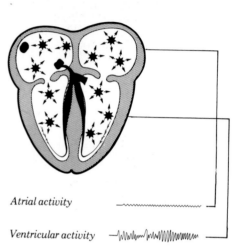

*Figure 88. Ventricular fibrillation*

*Atrial activity*

*Ventricular activity*

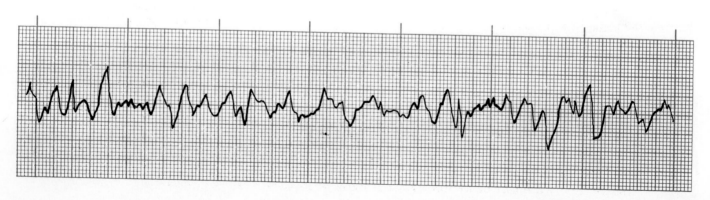

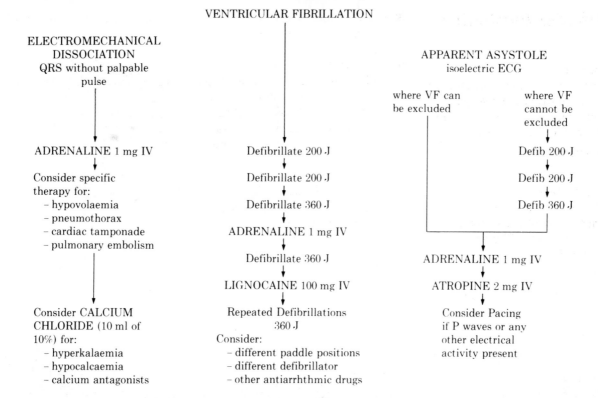

VENTRICULAR FIBRILLATION

ELECTROMECHANICAL
DISSOCIATION
QRS without palpable
pulse

APPARENT ASYSTOLE
isoelectric ECG

where VF can
be excluded

where VF
cannot be
excluded

ADRENALINE 1 mg IV

Defibrillate 200 J

Defib 200 J

Consider specific
therapy for:
  – hypovolaemia
  – pneumothorax
  – cardiac tamponade
  – pulmonary embolism

Defibrillate 200 J

Defib 200 J

Defibrillate 360 J

Defib 360 J

ADRENALINE 1 mg IV

Defibrillate 360 J

LIGNOCAINE 100 mg IV

ADRENALINE 1 mg IV

Consider CALCIUM
CHLORIDE (10 ml of
10%) for:
  – hyperkalaemia
  – hypocalcaemia
  – calcium antagonists

Repeated Defibrillations
360 J
Consider:
  – different paddle positions
  – different defibrillator
  – other antiarrhthmic drugs

ATROPINE 2 mg IV

Consider Pacing
if P waves or any
other electrical
activity present

Continue CPR for up to 2 min after each drug. Do not interrupt CPR for more than 10 sec except for defibrillation.
If an IV line cannot be established, consider giving double doses of adrenaline, lignocaine or atropine via an endotracheal
tube.

PROLONGED RESUSCITATION:
Give 1 mg ADRENALINE IV every 5 mins.
Consider 50 mmol SODIUM BICARBONATE (50 ml of 8.4%) or according to blood gas results.

# Ventricular standstill

*Figure 89. Ventricular standstill*

## Description
Total absence of ventricular activity. Atrial activity only is seen (Figure 89).

## ECG characteristic
■ Rate: ventricular – nil. Atrial rate may be normal
■ Rhythm: absent
■ P waves: normal
■ P–R interval: not identifiable
■ QRS complex: absent

## Clinical significance
Results in an absence of cardiac output, that is cardiac arrest.

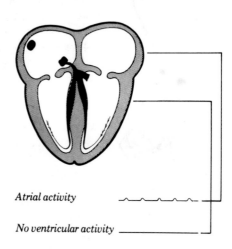

*Atrial activity*

*No ventricular activity*

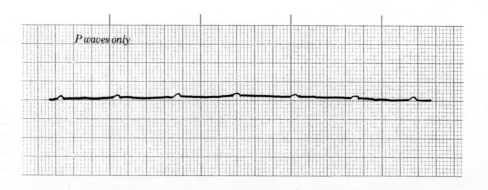

*P waves only*

# Ventricular flutter

This term may be used to describe a form of ventricular fibrillation which is seen as a series of large wave-like oscillations (Figure 90).

*Figure 90.*

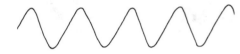

# Asystole

There is a total absence of myocardial activity resulting in a loss of cardiac output. Occasionally some bizarre-looking movement may be noted on the trace, at an extremely slow rate, often called *post-mortem artefact* or *dying heart syndrome* (Figure 91). Otherwise, all that can be seen is basically the isoelectric line on the monitor with some slight movement; rarely is it a perfectly straight line.

*Figure 91.*

If ventricular fibrillation can be excluded treatment will include Adrenaline, Atropine and possibly pacing. If ventricular fibrillation could not be excluded defibrillate at 200 J, 200 J, 360 J prior to starting drug therapy.

# Third-degree heart block

This is also known as complete heart block or complete atrioventricular dissociation.

**Description**
The A–V node does not conduct any impulses and therefore the atria and ventricles beat completely independently of each other. The S–A node continues to pace the atria but because the impulses are not conducted through the A–V node an ectopic focus in the ventricles takes over the control of the ventricles. If the ectopic focus is high up in the ventricles near the bundle of His the QRS complex may appear quite normal. If the ectopic focus is low in the ventricles the QRS complex may appear wide and bizarre. The P waves and QRS complexes have no relationship to each other, and the P waves are often lost in the QRS complexes. Occasionally a P wave may be seen prior to the QRS complex, but this is purely a coincidence, and the two have no

relationship to each other, and are completely dissociated (Figure 92).

### ECG characteristic
- Rate: atrial rate may be normal; ventricular rate may be 20–50 b.p.m.
- Rhythm: atria regular, ventricles usually regular
- P waves: normal, but may not be seen as they may be buried in the QRS complexes
- P–R interval: absent
- QRS complex: abnormal, the width and shape may vary depending upon exact focus.

### Clinical significance
The rhythm may be caused by damage to the A–V node, bundle of His or bundle branches (as in ischaemic heart disease or trauma) or increased parasympathetic tone. The ventricular rate is usually low with its associated lowering of cardiac output. The patient, therefore, will show the signs and symptoms of the lowered cardiac output; because of the slow rate ventricular dysrhythmias may appear, and there

is also the risk of deterioration to ventricular standstill.

### Treatment
If the rate is sufficient to maintain cardiac output little treatment may be required.

If the patient shows the signs and symptoms of the lowered cardiac output supportive therapy, such as oxygen therapy or entonox will be

required. An isoprenaline infusion may also be required – 4 mg of isoprenaline is added to 1000 ml of 5% dextrose and run through a Metriset, initially at 15 ml/hour (15 drops/min). The rate may be altered depending upon the ventricular response.

A pacemaker may also be inserted, temporarily for the emergency and, if necessary, permanently later.

*Figure 92.* Third-degree heart block (complete heart block)

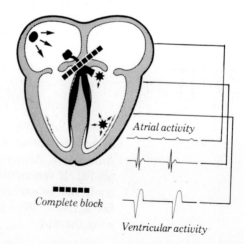

Atrial activity

Complete block

Ventricular activity

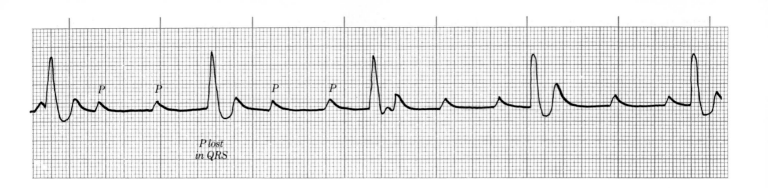

P lost
in QRS

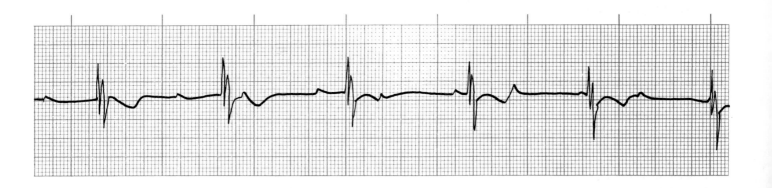

# Index

**A**

Abdomen   *21, 54–6, 62, 77*
Abdominal
  organs   *49*
  thrust   *55, 57, 60, 80*
Acidosis   *8, 10, 44, 88, 100, 104*
Adrenaline   *45, 46, 53, 88, 94*
  'surge'   *45*
Aerobic metabolism   *7*
Aftercare   *52*
Air 'sounds'   *37, 66, 72*
Airway   *1, 2, 8, 13–15, 17, 26, 33, 37, 38, 48, 49,*
    *52, 54, 56, 63, 65, 66*
  care   *1, 10, 12, 26, 34, 35, 36, 48, 73, 75, 80*
  clear the   *3, 13, 14, 26, 29, 56, 75, 76*
  obstruction   *3, 8, 9, 12–14, 16, 17, 23, 26, 31,*
    *38, 54, 62, 63, 77, 80*
  resistance   *16*
Alcohol   *77*
Alkalosis   *44*
Alternating current (AC)   *40*
Alveolar damage   *48*
Alveoli   *2, 4, 5, 7*
Alveolus   *4*
Ambu
  compact resuscitator   *34*
  resuscitator – baby model   *83*
  suction booster   *29, 30*
  suction 'pump'   *27*
Aminophylline   *94*
Amiodarone   *47*
Anaerobic metabolism   *7, 10*
Anaesthesia   *43, 66*
Analgesia   *47, 52, 94*
Anaphylactic reaction   *9*
Anoxia   *79*
Antecubital fossa   *44*
Anxiety   *45, 94*
Aorta   *5–7*
Aortic valve   *5–7*
Artefact   *39, 43*

Arteries   *5*
Artificial ventilation   *12, 15, 17, 19, 20, 22, 23,*
    *26, 34, 36, 44, 50, 51, 53, 54, 67, 72, 75, 76, 79*
Asphyxia   *76*
Asthma   *9*
Asystole   *38, 40, 41, 43, 46, 47, 50, 87, 88, 90,*
    *109*
Atherosclerosis   *48*
Atlanto-occipital joint   *67*
Atrial
  damage   *96*
  dysrhythmia   *89, 96*
  ectopics   *89, 96, 97*
  fibrillation   *89*
  flutter   *89*
Atrioventricular block   *47*
Atrioventricular node   *98, 109, 110*
Atrium   *5–7*
Atropine   *45, 47, 88, 92, 94*
  resistant bradycardia   *46*

**B**

Back blows   *58, 59, 61, 62*
Bag/valve/mask unit   *34, 35, 67, 82, 83*
Bag/valve unit   *36–8, 66, 72, 77*
β-blocker   *96, 98*
Bicuspid valve   *5, 6*
Blood
  gas analysis   *44, 50, 52, 88*
  pressure   *46, 92, 94, 104*
Body core temperature   *77–9*
Brachial pulse   *84*
Bradycardia   *47, 87, 88, 92*
Brain   *1, 5, 8, 18, 38, 53*
  damage   *1, 10, 50, 52, 79*
Breathing   *4, 12, 14, 15, 17, 33, 50, 52, 63, 65,*
    *77, 81, 78*
Bretylium   *47*
Bronchi   *3–5, 9*
Bronchioles   *4, 9*
Bronchiole, terminal   *4*
Bronchitis   *9*

Bronchodilators *47*
Bronchus *3, 4, 72, 77*
Brook airway *33*
Buddy treatment *78*
Bundle
  branch block *98*
Bundle of His *109, 110*
Burns *9, 42*

## C

'Café coronary' *54*
Calcium
  carbonate *47*
  chloride *45-7, 88*
Cannula *44, 88*
Capillaries *5*
Carbon dioxide *4, 5, 7*
  assessment of *5*
  high *5*
Carbon monoxide *9, 10*
Cardiac arrest *3, 7-9, 11, 25, 38, 40, 44, 52-4,
    59, 67, 75, 77, 90, 106, 108*
  causes of *8, 38, 52, 80*
  diagnosis of *10*
  diagnosis of type of *38*
  effect of *10*
  signs of *10*
  treatment of *10*
Cardiac function *48*
Cardiac massage, open chest *18*
Cardiac output *8, 16, 19, 20, 24, 25, 38, 41, 43,
    46, 49, 77, 87-90, 94, 98, 100, 104, 106, 109, 110*
Cardiac rhythm *38, 41, 43, 46, 89*
Cardiac tamponade *9*
Cardiogenic shock *47, 52*
Cardiopulmonary resuscitation *1, 20, 38, 44,
    46, 48-50, 53, 54*
Cardiorespiratory arrest *9, 45, 47, 79, 80, 89*
Cardioversion, synchronised *43, 98*
Carotid
  artery *6*
  blood flow *19, 20, 46, 53*

pulse *10, 16, 20, 50, 84*
  sinus massage *98*
Carina *3, 4*
Central nervous system *9, 79*
Cerebral
  blood flow *46, 92*
  blood vessels *10, 46*
  circulation *8, 45, 92*
  hypoxia *92, 98*
  irritation *104*
  oedema *52*
Cerebrovascular disease *9*
Cervical
  spine *67*
  spine injury *48*
Chandra, N. *53*
Chemical agents *9*
Chemoreceptors *5*
Chest
  cavity *5, 22, 65*
  compression *19, 23-5*
  movement *16*
  pain *98*
  thrusts *59, 60, 80*
Child
  airway care in the *29, 31, 59, 80*
  external chest compression in the *84, 87*
  ratio of ECC to EAR in the *87*
  resuscitation of the *79*
  ventilation of the *81, 83*
Choking, treatment of *54, 62*
Chordae tendinae *7*
Circulation *12, 17, 18, 20, 46, 50, 52, 63, 84*
Circulatory collapse *20, 25, 44, 77, 78*
Cobb, Dr L.A. *19*
Compensatory pause *96, 100*
Complete
  atrioventricular dissociation *109*
  heart block *46, 47, 88, 90, 109-11*
Conduction system *9, 104*
Conductive gel *42*
Congestive cardiac failure *94, 100*

Conscious(ness) *2, 3, 10, 31, 33, 43, 52, 53, 54,
    89, 73, 78*
Cordilox *98*
Core temperature *77-9*
Coronary
  artery disease *53, 80*
  blood flow *46*
  vessels *46*
Corrosive(s) *9, 17, 76*
Cough
  CPR *53*
  reflex *76*
Criley, Dr J.M. *19, 53*
Cross-finger technique *13, 29*
Crush injury *9*
Crystalloid *44*
Cyanosis *10, 54*

## D

Death *1, 50, 54, 77, 104*
Defib-pads *42*
Defibrillation *19, 40, 42, 43, 49, 53, 87*
  of the infant/child *87, 88*
Defibrillator *36, 38, 40-3, 53*
  paddles *39, 40, 42, 43, 87, 88*
  stored energy *41*
Dentures *14*
Depolarisation *41, 102*
Dextrose solution
  50% *89*
  5% *44, 46, 47, 88, 110*
Diagnosis *10*
Diaphragm *5, 17, 18, 55, 56, 62*
  ruptured *9*
Digoxin *9, 46, 92, 94, 96, 98*
Direct current (DC) *40*
Disopyramide *47, 104*
Diuretics *47, 94*
Dobutamine *46*
Dopamine *46, 47, 89*
Drowning *38*

Drug
  administration  *44, 45, 88*
  overdose  *9, 87, 98, 100, 104*
Dying heart syndrome  *109*
Dysrhythmia  *9, 36, 38, 39, 43, 44, 50, 53, 78, 79, 89, 96, 98*
  simulator  *89*

**E**

Ectopic
  beat  *96*
  focus  *96, 106, 109*
Elective cardioversion  *98*
Electric shock  *40*
Electrical resistance  *42*
Electrocardiograph (ECG)  *39, 40, 43, 49, 87, 98*
  monitor  *36, 38-40, 43, 49, 50, 87, 89, 109*
  recognition  *89*
  The ECG – What does it tell?  *89, 90*
Electrocution  *8, 9, 38, 87*
Electrode gel  *42*
Electromechanical dissociation  *38, 40, 43, 46, 89*
Electrolyte imbalance  *87*
Endocardium  *7*
Endotracheal intubation  *36, 49, 66, 67, 75, 76, 81, 88*
  difficulties with  *67, 75*
  position for  *67*
  technique of  *36, 66-74*
Endotracheal route  *44-7, 88*
Endotracheal tube  *4, 20, 29, 30, 33, 36-8, 44, 53, 66, 71-3, 75, 76*
  sizes  *76, 77*
Entonox  *94, 98, 110*
Epiglottis  *2, 3, 70*
Expired air resuscitation (EAR)  *14, 15, 17, 20, 25, 33, 35, 48, 54, 63, 81*
  combined with external chest compression  *22*
External cardiac compression  *20*

External chest compression (ECC)  *12, 16, 18-20, 22-6, 35, 38-40, 42, 44, 46, 48, 50, 53, 56, 63, 85, 89*
  mistakes in  *24, 25*
External jugular vein  *44*
Eyelash reflex  *50*

**F**

Femoral pulse  *10, 20, 50, 84*
Fever  *94*
Fibrillation waves  *106*
Finger sweep  *13, 80*
First-degree heart block  *89*
Flail segment  *9*
Flecainide  *47*
Fluid replacement  *44*
Foreign body/material  *13, 55, 66, 73, 74*

**G**

Gardiner, J.  *89, 90*
Gas exchange  *4*
Gastric
  contents  *17, 23, 26, 30, 38, 48, 49, 63, 75, 76*
  distension  *17*
Guedel airway  *30*

**H**

Haemorrhage  *38, 94*
Haemothorax  *9*
Hand position  *20, 21, 25, 49, 56, 58*
Head
  injury  *9*
  tilt  *48, 67, 75, 80*
Heart  *5, 7, 9, 18, 19, 22, 24, 25, 40, 42, 79, 85*
Heart block
  1st degree  *89*
  2nd degree mobitz type 2  *90*
  3rd degree  *109-11*
Heart failure  *94, 96*
Heat loss  *77, 78*
Heimlich, Professor H.J.  *54*
Heimlich technique  *16, 54, 58, 59, 62*

Hepatic vein  *6*
High impulse cardiopulmonary resuscitation  *19, 20*
Hyperventilate  *17*
Hyperventilation  *48*
Hypoglycaemia  *89*
Hypotension  *47, 104*
  effects of  *92, 98*
Hypothermia  *50, 77*
  definition of  *77*
  effects of  *78, 79*
  treatment of  *78, 79*
Hypoxia  *7, 9, 10, 44, 46, 54, 67, 79, 80, 87, 92, 94, 100, 104*

**I**

IMS Min-i-jet system  *45*
Infant
  airway care in the  *29, 31, 59, 80*
  external chest compression in the  *84-6*
  ratio of ECC to EAR in the  *87*
  resuscitation of the  *79, 82*
  ventilation of the  *81-3*
Inferior vena cava  *6, 7*
Insect sting  *9*
Inspiration  *50*
Intercostal muscles  *5*
Internal defibrillation  *40*
Intracardiac route  *45, 89*
Intrathoracic structures  *49*
Intravenous
  cannulation  *49, 88*
  infusion  *44*
  route  *46, 47*
Introducer, endotracheal tube  *72*
Ischaemic heart disease  *9, 98, 100, 104, 110*
Isoelectric line  *109*
Isoprenaline  *45, 46, 88, 94, 110*

**J**

Jaw  *69*
Joules  *41-3*

Jugular vein  *6*
Junctional rhythm  *89*

**K**

Knickerbocker, C.G.  *19*
Koenig, Dr F.  *18*
Kouwenhoven, W.B.  *19, 40*

**L**

Lactic acid  *7*
Laerdal
  adult resuscitator  *34, 35*
  'jet sucker'  *26, 27*
  resuscitator – infant model  *83*
  suction unit  *28*
Laryngectomy  *16*
Laryngoscope  *29, 36, 66–75*
Larynx  *2, 3, 9, 70, 76*
Left ventricular failure  *94*
Lignocaine  *45, 47, 88, 100, 102, 104*
  side effects of  *47, 104*
Liver  *25, 60, 85*
Lung(s)  *3, 5, 7, 9, 16–18, 25, 37, 54, 66*

**M**

Magill intubating forceps  *36, 66, 72–4*
Mandible  *2*
Manikin, training  *25, 35, 36, 48, 66, 74, 79*
Metabolic rate  *79*
Mexiletine  *47, 104*
Millimole  *44*
Min-i-jet system  *45*
Mitral valve  *5–7*
Monitoring electrodes, ECG  *39, 40*
Mouth/nose  *2, 55, 68*
Mouth-to-mouth ventilation  *14–17*
Mouth-to-nose ventilation  *15, 17*
Myocardial
  blood flow  *46*
  contractibility  *46*
  depression  *47*
  infarction  *9, 38*
  irritability  *46, 47*
  ischaemia  *94, 98, 104*
Myocardium  *7, 41, 46, 89, 94*

**N**

Nasal cavity  *2*
Nasopharyngeal
  airway  *30, 33*
  suction  *29*
Nasopharynx  *2, 33*
Neck extension  *14, 16, 33–5, 48*
Neurological
  deficit  *79*
  function  *48*
Nose  *2, 16*

**O**

Observation  *52*
Obstruction  *55, 56, 59, 62*
Oesophageal
  disease  *76*
  gastric tube airway  *76*
  obturator airway  *75, 76*
  temperature  *77, 78*
Oesophagus  *2, 17, 37, 75, 76*
Organic heart disease  *96*
Oropharyngeal
  airway  *30–3, 38, 73, 80*
  suction  *31*
Oropharynx  *2, 29, 33, 38, 67, 73, 75*
Oxygen  *1, 4, 5, 7, 8, 18, 34, 35, 38, 43, 47, 52, 53, 79, 83, 92, 94, 98, 110*
  assess  *5*
  carrying capacity  *9*
  lack  *8, 10*
  low  *5*
  reservoir bag  *35*

**P**

Pacemaker  *46, 110*
Paediatric resuscitation  *79*
Pain  *94*
Papillary muscle  *7*

Parasympathetic effect  *92, 100, 104, 110*
Partial pressure – carbon dioxide  *7*
Partial pressure – oxygen  *7, 10*
Pericardium  *7*
pH  *44*
Pharynx  *29, 76*
Physio Control Lifepack 5  *38–40*
Pleura  *3, 5*
  parietal  *5*
  visceral  *5*
Pneumothorax  *9, 45*
Poisoning  *9, 50*
Portal vein  *6*
Post-arrest  *46, 47, 89*
Posterior pharyngeal wall  *30, 31*
Post-mortem artefact  *109*
Potassium, serum  *104*
Practolol  *98*
Precordial 'thump'  *25, 85*
Premature
  atrial contractions  *96, 97*
  beat  *100*
  ventricular contractions  *100, 101*
Primary resuscitation  *12, 35*
Procainamide  *47*
Prognosis  *52*
Prophylaxis  *51*
Propranolol  *92*
Pulmonary
  artery  *6, 7*
  embolism  *9*
  oedema  *52*
  valve  *6, 7*
  veins  *5–7*
Pulse  *10, 16, 20, 24, 25, 50, 78, 85, 98*
Pump failure  *104*
Pupils  *10, 50, 78*
P waves  *98, 109*
Pyruvic acid  *7*

**Q**

QRS complex  *98, 100, 109*

'Quick look' ECG monitoring  *39*

**R**

Rankin, S.J.  *19*
Recovery
  phase  *52*
  position  *14, 63–5*
Rectal temperature  *77, 78*
Reflex vagal stimulation  *98*
Regurgitation  *17, 20, 23, 38, 48, 49, 63, 75, 76*
Reheating
  active  *78, 79*
  passive  *78*
Renal
  artery  *6*
  vein  *6*
Repolarisation  *102*
Respiration  *7, 10, 50, 78*
  mechanics of  *5*
Respiratory arrest  *7, 8, 10, 11, 14, 67, 80*
  causes of  *8*
Respiratory function  *48*
Respiratory movement  *50*
'Resusci-Aide'  *33*
Resuscitation  *1, 8, 10, 12, 19, 20, 24, 35, 37, 39, 43, 44, 48, 49, 51, 52, 59, 77, 79*
  drugs  *45*
  of infants and children  *79*
  of the newborn  *79*
  timing of  *22*
Rewarming
  active  *78, 79*
  passive  *78*
Rib fractures  *9, 25, 48, 59*
Ribs  *5*
R-on-T
  phenomenon  *43*
  ventricular ectopics  *90, 102, 103*
R-R interval  *96*
Rudikoff, M.T.  *53*
R wave  *43, 102*

**S**

Safar, Dr P.  *53*
Scald(s)  *9*
Secondary measures  *26*
Second-degree heart block  *90*
Sedation  *43, 47, 52, 77*
Shivering  *77, 78*
Shoulder blades  *58, 61*
Sinoatrial node  *90, 92, 94, 98, 109*
Sinus
  arrhythmia  *89*
  bradycardia  *88, 89, 92, 93*
  rhythm  *89–91*
  tachycardia  *89, 94, 95*
Skin
  temperature  *77*
  resistance  *44*
'Sniffing the morning air' position  *67*
Soda lime canister  *79*
Sodium
  bicarbonate  *44, 45, 47, 88*
  chloride  *47*
'Space blanket'  *78*
Spinal
  column  *18, 19, 67*
  cord injury  *9, 48*
Status epilepticus  *9*
Sternal compression  *19, 20*
Sternum  *18, 19, 21, 22, 25, 42, 54, 56, 59, 62, 85*
Steroids  *47*
Stomach  *17, 20, 23, 38, 48*
Strangulation  *9*
Stress  *45*
Subclavian
  artery  *6*
  vein  *6*
Successful or?  *50*
Suction equipment  *17, 26, 30, 33, 66, 73, 76*
Suffocation  *9*
Superior vena cava  *6, 7, 19*

Supraorbital pressure  *98*
Supraventricular tachycardia  *43, 89, 98, 99, 104*
Suscardia  *46*
Sympathetic effect  *94, 98, 100, 104*
Synchronised mode  *43*

**T**

Tachydysrhythmia(s)  *46*
Teeth  *69, 70*
Temperature  *77, 78*
  regulation  *77*
Tendon reflexes  *78*
Tension pneumothorax  *9*
Tertiary measures  *36*
Tetanus  *9*
Third-degree heart block  *109–11*
Thoracic cavity  *5, 9*
Tissue
  necrosis  *88*
  perfusion  *92, 94, 98, 104*
Tongue  *2, 12, 14, 16, 17, 31, 32, 63, 68, 70, 71*
Total airway obstruction  *54*
Toxic gases  *9*
Trachea  *3, 5, 9, 18, 36, 54, 66, 67, 77*
Tracheostomy  *16*
Trauma  *7, 8, 10, 17, 51, 77, 110*
Tricuspid valve  *6, 7*
T wave  *43, 100, 102*

**U**

Umbilicus  *54, 56, 62*
Unconscious(ness)  *1–3, 8, 10, 12, 56, 63, 66, 73, 75–8, 104*
Uterus  *59*

**V**

Vagus nerve  *92*
Valium  *94*
Vallecula  *2, 70*
Veins  *5*
Venae cavae  *7, 44*

Ventilation
  artificial   *12, 15, 17, 19, 20, 22, 23, 26, 34, 36, 44, 50, 52, 53, 54, 67, 72, 75, 76, 79*
  bag and mask   *34, 79*
  equipment for   *34, 66, 79*
  mouth-to-mouth   *14-17, 76*
  mouth-to-mouth and nose   *17, 81*
  mouth-to-nose   *15, 17*
  mouth-to-stoma   *16*
Ventricle   *5-7*
Ventricular
  dysrhythmia   *41, 47, 87, 88, 92, 100, 102, 106, 110*

ectopics   *90, 100-2*
fibrillation   *19, 36, 38, 40, 41, 43, 46, 53, 78, 87, 90, 102, 104, 106, 107, 109*
fibrillation, coarse   *106, 107*
fibrillation, fine   *46, 88, 106, 107*
fibrillation threshold   *47*
filling time   *94*
flutter   *90, 109*
myocardium   *100, 102, 104, 106*
rate   *46, 98, 110*
standstill   *90, 108, 110*
tachycardia   *43, 87, 90, 98, 104, 105*

Verapamil   *47, 98*
Vertebral artery – basilar artery system   *48*
Vocal cords   *3, 36, 62, 66, 70, 71, 75*

**W**

Weisfeldt, M.L.   *53*

**X**

Xylocard, 2% and 20%   *47*

**Y**

Yankaur suction catheter   *29*